To Norwyn whose own
story is so inspiring —
Best wishes,
Sandra Fiser

A Change of Heart

Sandra Fiser with Tom Fiser

CROSSBOOKS
PUBLISHING

CrossBooks™
A Division of LifeWay
1663 Liberty Drive
Bloomington, IN 47403
www.crossbooks.com
Phone: 1-866-879-0502

First published by CrossBooks 5/19/2010

ISBN: 978-1-6150-7192-0 (sc)
ISBN: 978-1-6150-7193-7 (hc)

Library of Congress Control Number: 2010926382

Printed in the United States of America
Bloomington, Indiana

This book is printed on acid-free paper.

Dedication

To donor families, who out of their heartbreak and pain, give the gift of life.

Contents

Epigraph

Moreover, I will give you a new heart and put a new spirit
Within you; and I will remove the heart of stone from your flesh
And give you a heart of flesh.
And I will put My Spirit within you and cause you to walk
In My statutes, and you will be careful to observe My ordinances.
Ezekiel 36:26-27

Foreword

This is a book for everyone. It is an illness narrative that will touch the heart while giving insight into one family's challenge of devastating disease. The words and story will more generally, help everyone better manage the challenges of life. Scurrying through the busy days, weeks, months, and years of Sandra and Tom Fisers' busy lives we see a fascinating tale of love, faith, and redemption. From the perspective of patients it will chronicle the courageous path taken by a family with the difficulties the day presents. A failed business is trivial when compared to devastating disease. Their path is filled with pain, suffering and uncertainty. But mostly, love. It was a love of one another and love of their faith. It was an admirable love which was true and tested deeply and daily for years. It was a love that survived doubt and fear, and will give hope to all with difficult illness – and maybe even difficult relationships.

To a professional health care provider, the tale will tell the inside story of what being a helpless, completely dependent, yet utterly trusting patient means. It will make the physician, nurse, resident, fellow, custodian, and social worker reflect on their purpose. It will also show the foibles and hubris we in the profession sometimes exhibit. It is an eye opening tome and should make us all want to be better care givers. Hospital administrators will learn a bit more of the patient experience and that we aren't just responsible for performing miraculous surgical procedures. Rather, we must also pay attention to the soul of the patient and family. It will teach the real meaning of care and healing and, perhaps, cure.

We surely hear the voice of the patient in this book and it is pleading, praising, and touching. The story asks for forgiveness, understanding, and help as the patient moves through the heady world of heart transplantation at an internationally recognized academic medical center. The story also brings to us the challenges of the clinicians and all of the care givers to surpass the bounds of disease. We should take away some simple truths about how and why we talk to patients and their families and be forced to learn a better way. It will make some of us remember that compassion and gentle truth is the key to conversation with a patient.

The story should also be read by friends of the ill. One will see the remarkable effect that simple but loving expression and small favors have on a patient in difficult times. The role of dear friends, faith partners, and even casual acquaintances of the Fisers' are detailed and it reminds us that small tokens of care and concern go far to help the suffering on their journey. Often times this is more effective than the most powerful antibiotic.

The heart transplant fraternity is unique. Having faced death and pain and uncertainty squarely in the eye, patients with advanced heart failure cope with their illnesses in many ways. Often it is healthy and heroic and admirable. Sometimes it is not. The Fisers chronicle this passage sensitively and admirably. They detail the extraordinary challenge of being cooped up, often with a roommate that can be a challenge, in an environment where any vestige of privacy is discarded. Tied permanently to lifesaving infusions or mechanical circulatory sustenance machines, the patients wait fearfully until they either die, or are lucky enough to receive a donor heart in a dramatic operation. Fortunately most make it and the intervention is more often successful, than not. Patients bond with their health care providers, other patients, and even visitors, while roaming the sterile and cold confines of the hospital ward while pushing their wheelie poles decorated with dangling ministrations that sometimes come to look like a Christmas tree of sorts. Only a deep trust in someone, something, and some faith can sustain one during that travail, and we see that in this story. The love the Fisers shared, love of each other, love of their family, love of their friends, and love of their faith sustained them and this should give us all heart and hope. The group of inpatients awaiting the chance for a CHANGE OF HEART has, on occasion, been described as "the yacht club". It is not an exclusive fraternity that one should clamor to join. Thrown together by fate and ill fortune it is the ultimate emotional and physical stress test. The Fisers survived as a couple in love and in faith – sometimes challenged to the near break point. Many will discover an "ah ha" in this story, as they should.

And so in the end, this is a story about an illness, faith, love and redemption. Though the faith is Christian, the tenants are relevant to all. There is a pearl for everyone brave enough to digest this remarkable and remarkably well written story. It may be lifesaving and faith saving to some. Tom Fiser and his wife Sandra, and their family are heroes. A suffering patient once explained to me, after my telling her that she "was my hero," that being a hero simply meant you didn't let "folks know just how scared you really were." Enjoy the illness journey chronicle the hero and heroine Fisers have graciously, courageously, and fearlessly given us all.

James B. Young, M.D.
Professor of Medicine and Executive Dean
Cleveland Clinic Lerner College of Medicine
of Case Western Reserve University
George and Linda Kaufman Chair
Chairman, Endocrinology and Metabolism Institute
Cleveland Clinic

Preface

As believers in Jesus Christ Tom and I do not think God caused Tom's heart problems. We do believe that God used those problems and experiences to educate and influence Tom and me. We praise God for loving two flawed human beings enough to save them, even when they worked at cross purposes to the divine plan. Are we presenting ourselves as special? We are not. We do not know why God in His mercy guided us through this long and arduous journey, stationing the right people and events in place to work toward our successful end-but He did. We are convinced of this, and we humbly give Him thanks. Tom and I have researched more than twenty years of hospital records and physicians' notes in an attempt to be medically accurate while telling our story in layman's language. Our impressions of people and situations encountered along the way are written from our combined memories and journal notes. They are recounted as we remember them, not as fact. Writing *A Change of Heart* has been both painful and healing. It has required a level of transparency new to both of us. We hope that telling our story will encourage others who find themselves struggling against seemingly overwhelming odds. May it remind them that they are not alone.

Acknowledgments

We would like to thank Bette Callaway, Nancy Shuffield, Tad Fiser, and Leigh Compton for their willingness to read and re-read the drafts of this work. Their insight, encouragement, and support of our efforts were priceless.

A host of friends, family, and neighbors, the congregations and staffs of Pulaski Heights Baptist Church, Pulaski Heights Methodist Church, and Fellowship Bible Church, Dr. John Kagy, Dr. James Metrailer, Dr. Charles Watson, Dr. Scott Davis, the nurses and staff of St. Vincent's Infirmary, and of the Cleveland Clinic, our Supper Club, and *The Board* have been more than kind and generous over the past decades. We thank them, and we consider ourselves blessed to have had them in our lives.

A very special acknowledgment is due Dr. Andrew Kumpuris and Dr. Michael Bauer who with God's grace kept Tom's heart functioning for twenty years, and Dr. James Young who facilitated Tom's evaluation prior to his becoming a patient of the Cleveland Clinic Transplant Program. We humbly thank Dr. Young as well for his graciousness in writing the foreword for *A Change of Heart*.

Finally, words fail when we think of thanking those who have lived this adventure with us. Leigh Fiser Compton and Samantha, Tad and Laura Fiser, Ben, Hannah, Claire you have loved us and supported us; you've cried with us and laughed with us and prayed with us and for us. Brian and Zachery Compton, we welcome you to the rest of the adventure. We love you all with a mighty love.

1

Death Sentence

Tom and I sat in the small examining room-a place much too familiar to us. Outside, it was an Arkansas autumn day, hot and humid. Inside, an air conditioner whirred in spite of the fact that the calendar said it was October. Fall can be like that in our state-either dry and thirsty or buried in sodden pods of humidity that leave you dragging from chore to chore, seeking relief indoors or beside one of our lakes or streams.

On the wall was a print, the kind once popular with lovers of Americana, of a man on horseback in front of a ramshackle, frontier, mountain cabin. The rider was visiting with a disreputable-looking mountaineer seated on the cabin's front porch. The print was titled "The Arkansaw Traveler." I had never liked it-or at least I did not like the picture I perceived it presented of our citizenry as ignorant and slothful. Bookcases filled with medical books studied by our physician and his father before him lined another wall. On the other side of the room was a small window looking out on another medical office building. There was not much to see and we had certainly seen it all before. Tom sat on an examining table that was on its second generation of patients and physicians. This was a utilitarian room-a room that was made for bare-bones pronouncements of good or ill health. It lacked the stylish accouterments and soft lighting of this equivocating age when hard sayings are often couched in soft phrases.

Tom and I talked, speaking of this and that and nothing. We stared out the glass as if the small window opened on a lovely vista. I studiously read and re-read the titles of the thick medical tomes in their cases. We sat in silence, each lost in thoughts that would not bear voicing.

The door opened. Dr. Drew entered briskly. We exchanged brief pleasantries before he told Tom to unbutton his shirt. Putting his stethoscope to his ears, he listened to Tom's heart. When he had removed the stethoscope from his ears, the three of us made small talk as Dr. Drew thumbed through the voluminous chart that held more than twenty years of Tom's heart history. I am sure Dr. Drew did more, listening to Tom's back, prodding his stomach, and conducting a routine examination. Excusing himself, chart under his arm, Dr. Drew left the examining room, shutting the door behind him. He said he would only be a minute.

Tom buttoned his shirt. We discussed the day's remaining chores. I smiled brightly, knowing from past experience that this was expected. Beneath the unforgiving light in this medical cubicle Tom looked gray, his face lined. Behind my smile, the nagging harpies of fear circled my soul like so many buzzards. Outwardly Tom wasn't fazed by this visit. It was simply an interruption in the pattern of his life.

In fact, we were here in this place again less than two years after Tom's fifth heart surgery. My husband remembers thinking that the results of this visit to the cardiologist would be similar to the results of visits that had gone before. Dr. Drew would outline the problem and present the plan for its solution. Tom would screw up his courage, saying, "Let's get this over with, doc," and they would-just as they had through five previous surgeries and countless procedures. With Tom, it was always "get it over with, and get on to the next event." He allowed few chinks in the armor of his positive, can-do attitude. I was always the quivering mass of uncertainties and fears hiding behind the requisite smile.

Neither Tom nor I was prepared for what came next. Dr. Drew returned to our room, sat down, and said, "Mr. Fiser, there is nothing more I can do. You are in heart failure, and without a heart transplant, you most likely will die." The words on the page are cold; uttered aloud they were filled with regret.

As I stared at him, Tom's demeanor registered disbelief. How could the man who for twenty years had been the go-to-guy say there was nothing more he could do? Tom struggled to resurrect the smile of bravado with which he had faced the previous five surgeries. Tiny and weak, it tugged at the corners of his lips-then slipped stillborn from his face. The mixture of denial and positive thinking that he had concocted to help him feel in control during his previous illnesses and surgeries dissipated in that moment.

While I had faced Tom's bouts with heart disease with more realism (he called it pessimism) than he, I had never expected to hear the physician say nothing more could be done. I was, for the moment, too stunned to cry. I had imagined massive, murdering coronary attacks-but not a quiet sentence regretfully uttered.

Trying to absorb the enormity of what lay ahead, Tom and I listened as Dr. Drew began outlining my husband's immediate care and our options. In my imagination, I see us both gasping for air in an oxygen-starved environment, divers who have descended to the limit of their lung capacity before surfacing in a dark and choppy sea. The doctor's words swirled and spiraled in dizzying array as we clutched at them. Immediately there would be changes in medication to ease the load on Tom's worn-out heart muscle. Prescriptions were written, signed, and placed in Tom's hand. Arrangements were made for him to attend a heart failure clinic at one of the local hospitals. Dr. Drew said we could then make plans to have Tom evaluated for a heart transplant. The silence was absolute. *Transplant*-the word was a giant rock dropped into our shared air space, and the ripples from it washed over us in waves.

The doctor, seemingly unaware of this disruption, reminded us that a small but successful transplant program operated at one of the hospitals in our city, or there were larger, successful programs in a number of other cities around the country. My ears had closed after the phrase *heart transplant*. What an awesome, awful, hopeful, discouraging utterance. Tom's mind and emotions were in overload as well as mine. Dr. Drew continued, telling us that at one of those larger centers he had a good friend from his medical school days who worked as head of the heart transplant program. He would be willing to ask him if Tom met the criteria for evaluation by that hospital.

Tom's answer was swift and negative. "No." Tom said he would not consider a transplant. He had burdened the family enough. He thought of the time, money, and strength this would require-not only from the two of us, but from our entire family. He would not put us all through this. Tom could call to mind only the news stories of one of the earlier heart transplant patients who had not lived to leave the hospital.

I grabbed the nearest life vest in the roiling waters of my fears-prayer, silent, and swift, and without a doubt, incoherent. My emotions were so raw and my mind such a jumble that my silent prayers were those wordless groans that we are told the Spirit brings to order before the throne of the Father. In tears, struggling for composure, I begged Tom to consider the transplant option, to discuss it with our family, and to pray about his decision. I reminded him that my cousin had, several years earlier, received a heart enabling him to live to see his son grow up. Although their diagnoses and their ages were different, I argued that a transplant might also work for Tom. I pleaded with him not to shut any doors. I assured him that the children and I would abide by his decision, whatever it was. God surely gave me those words and the strength to say them. I said it and meant it-but finding the strength to see it through could not come from me as my mind and my emotions churned out of control.

We must have discussed at least a few other things with Dr. Drew before leaving his office. Tom does not remember, nor do I. We left the examining room, walked through the office waiting area, and stepped out into a world where nothing had changed. There should have been dark clouds and violent winds to match our emotional and spiritual upheaval, but there were none. It was not Cecil B. DeMille, but God, directing our day-as He would all the days to come.

2

The Road to Infarction

Flash back twenty years to another October day when the air was clear and crisp, and the red and gold leaves of the southern hardwoods were jewel-like. Tom and Tad, our fifteen-year-old son, were on the road to Tom's brother Robert's hunting and fishing camp on the banks of the Ouachita River in south Arkansas. Roughly built and deep in the woods, the camp stood on a high bluff that had once been home to Confederate gun emplacements. My brother-in-law's cabin was first in a line of three spaced along the top of the bluff, each about fifty yards from the other. The timber, land, and the cabins had all belonged to one family until Robert had endeared himself to them through his friendship with one of their sons. The family patriarch and Robert visited often over the years. In time the old man, who looked on Robert as a son, deeded the cabin and its acre and a half of ground to him.

Reaching the camp about dusk, the guys made a campfire, ate, and planned the details of their weekend. There would be an early morning tramp through the woods stalking the stealthy squirrels. They planned to hunt a while before rigging a way to plug in an ancient television set outside the cabin. Getting the television into the outdoors was the key to enjoying simultaneously a campfire, the sights and smells of the woods, and the premier rivalry of the 1981 Southwest Conference-the Arkansas Razorbacks and the Texas Longhorns. With visions of squirrels and Razorbacks dancing in their dreams, the men fell asleep.

The Saturday morning dawn, viewed through the colorful canopy of leaves, was splendid. Our son and his uncle, the serious hunters of the trio, set out through the woods. Tom walked alone at a leisurely pace, up and down some small hills, more interested in enjoying the freedom of the forest than in finding and shooting a squirrel. Ambling along, he became aware of a slight tingle in his left arm and chest. Tom, in his early forties, never thought that it might be his heart. The sensation persisted without worsening. It reminded Tom of the burning sensation he had felt in his chest as a teenager when he ran wind sprints; he assumed he must be more out of shape than he had realized. Stopping, he lowered himself to the ground and leaned against a tree waiting for some hapless squirrel to wander by. As he sat there, the burning in his chest stopped; the tingling in his arm stopped. He felt fine and walked back to the camp without further problems. Since the pain had disappeared, Tom erased it from his mind, neither thinking more about it, nor telling his camp mates about the incident.

Lunch and a second short hunt were unremarkable either for strange tingling sensations, or for opportunities to shoot. It didn't matter to Tom. He was relishing the momentary respite from the pressures of running a small business. As the business grew he was finding himself wearing all the hats-CEO, chief researcher, quality control officer, sales manager, technical service. He was *the man*. A month earlier he had answered an emergency call to a job site where the slip of a tool (as he modified a piece of fiberglass pipe) narrowly missed lacerating the tendons and nerve bundles in his right hand. Tom talked about finding qualified help, not that he was not qualified himself after working for years in similar positions for a large manufacturing company. The truth was Tom liked being in control; he worked best under stress. When the time was right he would consider relinquishing some of the load, but the time was not right. Deadlines motivated Tom. The time in the woods was great, but come Monday morning he would be back in the ring ready to fight any and all company problems. He was at the top of his game. Medication controlled the high blood pressure Tom had developed while in graduate school. The Type II diabetes, discovered in a routine physical the previous year, was more or less controlled by diet when he chose to follow it. He had tested *barely* diabetic-borderline-there was no danger in that.

The trio of luckless hunters gathered, minus any game, back at the camp to snack and to watch the game. To their delight (and that of every other citizen of Arkansas) the Razorbacks trounced the Texas Longhorns.

The guys whooped, rejoiced and called the Hogs; any squirrel lingering in the surrounding woods fled the commotion.

Reliving every glorious moment of their team's victory, Tom, Robert, and Tad built another campfire, and cooked a victors' feast of grilled steak with all the trimmings, including my brother-in-law's signature steak sauce. The men, appetites satisfied, were lingering around the campfire when the neighbors in the next cabin called out to them. It was the habit of this large group of family and friends to meet most weekends in one of their cabins for food, usually venison and greens, and conversation. The brothers and Tad joined them; swapping tales and tidbits of local news for hours as the crowd gathered in the house grew and spilled onto the front porch. As the night deepened Tom, tired and in a reflective mood, ambled alone back to Robert's place. Poking the waning campfire back to life, he sat at ease staring into the flames until Robert and Tad returned. Tad wanted popcorn cooked over the fire and doused with hot sauce. Snacking on that, Tom and Robert regaled Tad with tales of their childhood on a small dairy farm. As the fire's embers died, so did the sounds of conversation from the cabins down the bluff. There was a distinct chill in the air. The hunters burrowed into sleeping bags they had spread on bunks within the half-screen walls of the cabin. Tom recalls no pain or discomfort that night, only the soothing night sounds of the woods lulling him to sleep.

Sunday morning dawned with the perfection of a travelogue description of an autumn campout in the woods. Robert had the campfire banked, and a pot of coffee boiling on it as Tom awoke. Fortified by their first cup of the black, steaming liquid, the guys cooked, and enjoyed a huge, outdoor breakfast of biscuits, bacon, and scrambled eggs. After tidying their campsite, the men set out on a final hunt before returning to the city. Again, the serious hunters, Robert and Tad, chose one trail, and Tom walked another. He had not hiked far into the forest when the tingling in his chest and arm returned with more intensity than he had experienced the previous day.

Cocooned in the myth of his own invincibility, Tom had no thought that this pain might be the result of anything more than the cold October air hitting his lungs-lungs he had recently deprived of their two-pack-a-day habit. Two weeks earlier Tom had given up his cigarettes cold turkey. We were spending the weekend in a lakeside condominium with close friends. As both men puffed one cigarette after another, the air in the room grew heavy with smoke. Sunlight coming through a large window emphasized the cloud they had created-one too thick to ignore. Janet and I commented on how much the guys smoked; we had been doing that for some time, but it was the visual image of that cloud that made Tom quit. Both men squelched their cigarettes, Tom for good, and James for a while.

Increasingly uncomfortable as the strange tingling sensations continued in his chest and his arm, Tom did not want to spoil the remainder of the outing for Tad and Robert. He decided to return early to the city. Tracking them down, Tom explained that he was tired of hunting and that he was returning to the city, but that he would leave our son to come home later in the afternoon with his uncle. Convinced that the pain was insignificant and that it would soon pass, he never mentioned the tingling and slight pain in his chest and arm. Tom packed his gear and started the two-hour drive home alone.

Setting the cruise control, he rolled down the highway toward home, and the strange sensation in his chest and arm disappeared. Tom's thoughts turned to work-related items-what needed to be shipped to maintain receivables; an employee who needed counseling regarding attendance. There were also family activities to be considered in the coming week-a high school football game with his son, a Halloween party for his sixth-grade daughter. He had a lot of ground to cover in the next seven days; as always, he was confident he could do it. Once home, Tom shared stories about the weekend with his wife and daughter. He told them about the great meals they'd cooked over the campfire, the beauty of the woods, and the lack of squirrels. He did not mention the burning in his chest, or the tingling in his left arm.

Monday morning, like most work days then, started with a roar rather than with a quiet time with God. Tom, an early riser, wanted time alone in his office before the phone and the factory challenges intruded. The burning was back in his chest and his left arm tingled as he showered, shaved, and dressed. He endured it, he ignored it, and he did not mention it to his wife before going out the door. As the day wore on, the burning sensation in Tom's chest became constant. Finally he told his brother, Robert, who worked with him in the business, that he had this "kind of strange feeling" in his chest; he was developing a chest cold from his outing in the woods. Robert, more cautious than his older brother, commented, "Could be your heart." Tom was incredulous-*Heart problems?* What nonsense! He was barely forty-three for God's sake! Turning on his heel, Tom stalked off, ignoring Robert's suggestion that he should have his heart checked. As in so many instances in this journey, it was for Tom's sake that God dealt patiently and gently with procrastination and prodigal ways.

As we drove that evening to a nearby town for our son's football game, Tom remained silent about the uncomfortable burning sensation in his chest, and the intermittent tingling in his left arm. He seemed a little more uptight, a little more frustrated by traffic than was usual, but I chalked it up to pressures at the plant. As Tom moved frenetically from engagement to engagement, he was often visibly and verbally frustrated

Early in the cold and windy first quarter of the football game, Tom and our daughter, Leigh, walked a hundred yards or so from the bleachers up a steep little incline to the concession stand to buy some coffee and hot chocolate. As he walked, Tom felt a jolt of pain in his chest. Gulping in cold air, he began to cough, which he continued to do as he paid for the drinks and returned to the stands. As he reached our seats, Tom said to me that he thought he had picked up a cold when he went hunting, and that his chest felt tight. He did not mention the tingling in his arm. He continued coughing between sips of hot coffee, and when Leigh and I voiced our concern, he grudgingly allowed that the discomfort in his chest might be the onset of pleurisy. He said emphatically that he did not want to leave the game; he did not want to be questioned about his self-diagnosed pleurisy. As we sat through the remaining quarters in the wind-swept stands, if Tom, coughing and unapproachable, had any doubts about his heart, he refused to face them. There was no room in his game plan for a sick heart.

Driving home after the game, the pain in Tom's chest lessened as the car grew warmer. His cough quieted. We rode without much conversation. Once Tom was in his warm bed, he slept well, coughing only sporadically throughout the night. The next morning as he prepared to go to work, I questioned Tom again about his cough and the tightness in his chest. "Pleurisy," he insisted as he shut the back door on his way to the car. I was left with the breakfast dishes, a nagging but as yet unidentified worry and a car pool run to make before I joined Tom at our business where I worked part-time as an office manager.

A couple of days passed with Tom coughing, and me expressing my concern about the cough. Tom made it clear that he saw my expressions of concern as nagging, raising the tension in our lives. Thursday, five days after the onset of the tingling in his arm and the tightness in his chest, Tom and I left the factory in the early afternoon to run an errand. We drove across town to the Farmers' Market to buy a dozen small pumpkins for a Halloween party our eleven-year-old Leigh was having on the weekend.

As Tom loaded the heavy sack of small gourds into the back of our station wagon I saw him wince, and heard the sharp intake of his breath when an unexpected pain hit him in the chest. I saw his reaction. Since his pain was visible he had little wiggle room for denial, but deny he did. An intense battle of wills ensued. I wanted to drive; Tom would not relinquish the keys. I insisted that Tom see our family doctor right away. Tom countered that he had no appointment. We sparred throughout the ride across the river and west toward home. As we neared our neighborhood, Tom agreed to see the doctor "in order to get some peace and quiet." Later Tom would admit that he had suffered chest pain the entire afternoon.

Pulling off the street, Tom found a parking place and walked angrily to our doctor's office with me hurrying to keep step. He was still protesting that it was unlikely that he would be seen without an appointment when the nurse appeared. Tom told her that I was overreacting to some pain he had been experiencing the past few days. He reiterated that the pressure in his chest was *pleurisy,* but he added that he'd had an intermittent tingling in his left arm for the past five days. The nurse whisked him into an examining room. Still protesting, Tom was attached to an electrocardiogram machine. Dr. Johns entered the room, questioned Tom, listened to his chest, heard the assertions of pleurisy, and read the EKG.

After the nurse disconnected him from the machine's electrodes, Tom reclaimed his shirt. Just as he began buttoning it Dr. Johns came back into the room and said, "Go directly to the hospital and let your wife drive." My husband stood with his shirt half on, dumbstruck for only a second before recovering his voice. He started to argue but Dr. Johns, a quiet, no-nonsense sort, stated again, this time more firmly, that Tom was to proceed to the hospital.

In total denial about what his symptoms might portend, Tom did not like having his plans thwarted. He had expected to see the physician, get a prescription for his *pleurisy* and go home. At most he might agree to a day or two in bed. Tom fumed, wrapping himself ever tighter in his security blanket of denial. Dr. Johns, ignoring the stormy expression on Tom's face, stared straight into his eyes and said, "I think you may have had a heart attack." Those words-*heart attack*-blew like a brisk, cold wind through the examining room leaving Tom naked before a very large truth that he refused to grasp; he was neither invincible nor in total control. Just as Adam had grabbed a fig leaf to hide his nudity from God, Tom, striped of his invincibility, wrapped himself in a security blanket of denial. In an attempt to maintain control he grabbed reasons why he could not go straight to the hospital. In those pre-cell-phone days there were calls he had to make. We needed to arrange for someone to be at home for our daughter after school. He needed his razor and pajamas. Finally, Tom sputtered that the trip to the hospital was needless. Faced with an implacable physician and a wife he saw as badgering, Tom consented to compromise. I could drive; we would circle by home for his pajamas and razor, and to call my parents to ask them to drive to our house to stay with Leigh when she came in from school. Our son, who had turned sixteen and was driving, had after school activities and wouldn't be home until later. Tom was still blustering about the inconvenience of this trip to the hospital as we left the doctor's office. I was absorbing the name of the worry that had nibbled at my peace for a week—*heart attack*.

3

Time Out

Tom and I were busy, not bad people. We attended church regularly, worked with the youth group; we valued family and friends. Our goals were admirable. We wanted to give our children every possible opportunity. We were in control, bothering God only when we felt He needed a little prodding to see things our way. We called ourselves good Christians.

God, having done His own prodding, and having found us reluctant to reconsider our priorities, called our first time out and pulled Tom from the game. He could have called the game. I want to repeat that we do not think God caused Tom's heart attack-not then, nor in the episodes that would follow. Tom's genes predisposed him to heart disease; his choices exacerbated his disease. We do not believe that our loving God sets out to harm His children. We do believe that He holds us accountable for our choices, and that those choices have consequences. We made the choices; we suffered the consequences. God used the circumstances to teach us, to mold us, to grow us, and to draw us closer to Him.

I have a penchant for speed when driving even under ordinary circumstances so we reached the hospital in record time. Tom assured me that if he actually had any heart problems, he would not have survived the ride. He refused a wheelchair, entering the emergency room under his own power, proclaiming all the while that he would be examined, released and sent home in short order. In short order he was sent, not home, but to the cardiovascular intensive care unit. I remained at the admissions desk filling out forms.

There is strength in numbers; separated we both felt uneasy and unsure in the unexpected situation in which we found ourselves; Tom blustering with bravado while I became increasingly anxious. Tom was being undressed, robed in a hospital gown that opened north and south, and hooked to monitors that banked both sides of the narrow and uncomfortable looking hospital bed while I registered him as a patient. He was in a glass room a little larger than a good-size broom closet. He had no privacy. Tom was indignant, still holding the probability that he'd had a heart attack at bay. My husband wondered what was taking so long and why I had not yet joined him.

The reality of our situation was sinking in as I filled out forms downstairs in admissions. I found a pay phone, called Tad's school, and asked the priest who was his principal to prepare our son for what had happened. I called our house to be certain that my parents had arrived to be there for the kids when they did get home. I put another coin in the phone and called Tom's parents. I boarded an elevator; got off on the right floor, and found the ICU where a nurse took me to Tom's cubicle-*cell*-he called it. I did the necessary chores in a fog. Our daughter, Leigh, says that during this time in our lives I functioned on auto pilot a good bit of the time. No doubt she is correct. Thinking back, what is amazing is that I expected our barely sixteen-year-old son to drive himself safely home after being told his father had suffered a heart attack, and had been hospitalized. To me, that is a clear indication that I was so overwhelmed I wasn't thinking clearly, or that I had a lot of confidence in Tad's maturity-probably it was a bit of both.

In 1981 the cardiovascular intensive care regimen at this particular hospital was strict. Tom's glass room had no television, no telephone, and he received no newspaper. On his wall Tom had a large, schoolroom-type clock and a calendar from which a page could be ripped day by day. The hospital was run by a religious order; there was a crucifix on the wall. There was a sink for the physician and nurses, a straight chair for one visitor at a time (the patient was bed bound), a rolling, adjustable tray which held a water pitcher and a glass with a straw. In addition there were the machines, tubes, bright lights, pumps, and whatever other machinery might be needed to sustain life in a broken heart. It was a sterile, forbidding and crowded environment. Visitors were allowed four times a day. Only persons over the age of twelve could visit. The rules were vigorously enforced.

Memories of our first time out flood back in a helter-skelter fashion, but two facts are paramount. Tom did not respond well to this enforced isolation from his family, his business, his world. He was frustrated and frightened. After more procedures than he can count, five heart surgeries, and a heart transplant, Tom still remembers that first night in CICU as the worst night of his life. He likens it to how he thinks a prisoner of war might feel, stripped of his identity, restrained in a foreign environment, unable to communicate with loved ones, held against his will by people he did not know or trust. To recall it is difficult for him. I quickly learned that my role was to curb my emotions, to study my words, to dress well, to put on make-up, and to smile as if everything was fine.

Passing the nurses' desk, I returned to a waiting room to count the hours until I would be allowed to see Tom again. Before many minutes passed, a hostess brought word that my father was on his way to the hospital to wait with me for news about the extent of the damage done to Tom's heart. I started walking through the hospital to meet my dad. My emotions were in turmoil, and I had not paid attention to where I was going when I had come to Tom's room from admissions. Under the best of circumstances, having always needed a map and a large dose of luck to get from point A to point B, I got lost in the halls of the hospital. A kind nun found me in the hallway, a woman in her late thirties, crying and saying that I could not find my daddy. The last time I had done that was in Hudson's Department Store in Detroit when I was seven! Together the nun and I found my dad.

Our support group in the waiting room grew. Tom's parents came. I think it was my mother who brought our children to the hospital. Tad, at sixteen, was old enough to see his father at visiting hour; eleven-year-old Leigh was not. An empathetic CICU nurse, seeing how upset our daughter was, took her and her brother to see their father. She took them back immediately, and spent some time explaining all the tubes, buttons, and monitors to them as she allowed them a short visit with their dad. She waited while they each hugged Tom, and still trying to answer their questions, the nurse ushered Tad and Leigh back to the waiting room. We all had so many questions and so few answers.

The cardiologist, after examining Tom, came to speak with me. All he would say was that Tom's EKG indicated that there was a problem. He would not tell me what might be the extent of the damage to the heart or Tom's prognosis. He would only say that as other test results were available, we would discuss them. He spoke with a wisdom and professionalism that I had to learn to appreciate. Seeking any straw to clutch and dissatisfied with what seemed to me to be a vague answer, I called a cousin, a long-time family doctor in eastern Arkansas, to complain that I had to have answers in order to have hope. With the wisdom born of years of dealing with anxious families in similar situations, he responded none too gently that I had exactly what I needed, a fine and competent physician. He said that the physician would talk with me when he had something to talk about. No one, he said, had a crystal ball to look into to give me guarantees about the future. I cannot say that this truth did much to relieve my anxiety but it stopped my whining. I claimed to profess a faith that said only God knew and controlled the future, but I did not fully grasp that truth. If God loved us enough to die for us, He loves us enough to live with us through whatever may lie before us. I chose anxiety rather than grasping that in the uncertainty of life the one constant is God's love.

Visiting hours were over; I would not be allowed to see Tom before morning. The nurses would call if there was any change, and we lived less than twenty minutes from the hospital. I could not leave. I needed to be physically in the same building with Tom. Grandparents had taken the children home and were with them. I sat in the CCU waiting room, chilled by an unwelcome breeze each time a nearby outside door opened. I replayed the day's events in my mind trying to make sense of them. The door opened with another frigid blast and Margaret entered the waiting room. Margaret was a delightful older lady in our church, a strong believer, wife of a physician, and a champion of good causes, and cases others might consider hopeless or unworthy. We loved Margaret, and we loved reading all the bumper stickers that were plastered across the back of her station wagon proclaiming her causes. Bundled against the cold, Margaret walked toward me carrying a pot of yellow chrysanthemums which she put in my hands. The flowers were cheerful and Margaret's presence was comforting. She prayed that evening for Tom, for me, for the children, the doctors. Margaret was a prayer warrior and I knew if God heard anyone that evening, He heard Margaret. With a hug and a promise to keep praying, she left me clutching the pot of mums. Margaret was one of many comforters the Father provided for us over the years as He faithfully sent others to prop us up when we could not stand alone.

The volunteer hostess, another older woman, did not leave the waiting room as I had assumed she would, hurrying through the cold to get home before dark. She stayed and ministered quietly to those caught in this place of uncertainty. Dimming the lights, she brought pillows and blankets as most of us tried to find a comfortable way to sleep in our chairs. I sat rigidly in my chair with Margaret's pot of mums resting in my lap. I've never found it easy to fall asleep; when my body slows, it seems my mind speeds up. That evening was no exception. As the hostess returned to her desk, she offered to place my potted plant on it. I relinquished the mums. Setting them between us she smiled and, speaking softly, told me who she was, and why she chose the late shift in the waiting room. She was a woman of faith, a member of the church that supported this hospital. She was a widow who had enjoyed a full and good life. She enjoyed helping others. Not many volunteers wanted to be at the hospital into the evening hours, but since no one waited dinner for her at home, she was able to give back to others in this way and at this time. Additionally, her only son had been a practicing physician at this hospital before his untimely death. She felt closer to him volunteering in this place where he had worked. She asked about my family, especially my children. She expressed confidence that my husband would improve saying that she would pray for him. We talked quietly until she left the hospital around nine o'clock. I don't remember that I slept, but I do remember that I was more calm and at peace. God sent a caring stranger who offered me encouragement.

I prayed during Tom's first hospitalization. I am sure Tom prayed as well, although I do not remember that we discussed prayer or spiritual things. Our conversations were stilted, banal. I smilingly assured Tom that all was well at home and at the business. He solemnly told me he was okay. The chasm of unasked questions and unexpressed concerns was wide and deep. By trying so hard to protect each other, we became isolated from each other, undermining the mutual support we could have provided. I did pray though. I prayed scared, I prayed bullet prayers, and at times it felt as if I prayed without ceasing. God probably thought I prayed without ceasing as I clattered on with my laundry list of wants, stopping only rarely to listen for any small, still voice of guidance and comfort from the Spirit. God could have roared in the voice of a lion, and I might not have heard unless He had said what I wanted Him to say.

The cardiologist told us that the cardiac enzymes and some other markers did indicate that Tom had suffered a myocardial infarction-a heart attack. Tom counted the clock's mechanical jerks as it moved moment by moment through each slow day. He anticipated the ripping of each day's page from the wall calendar. I juggled lots of balls during the day running from home, to the factory, to the school, to the hospital, and home again. More than once when the children were in their beds, I locked my bathroom door and cried. In one particularly bleak bout with fear and self-pity, I even cursed God. For a Bible-belt girl raised in a Southern Baptist church, there was nothing more shockingly awful, or condemning of my own soul that I could have done. For years carrying a huge guilt that was debilitating to my relationship with the Father, I told no one what I had done. I also, in ways that I did not understand, resented Tom for having a heart attack. Likewise that relationship suffered. Those two things were among the most difficult burdens that I had to bear. Eventually, I did understand that while it was self-centered, and rooted in fear of the unknown, my resentment of Tom for having the heart attack was not unusual. It took longer to realize that though my angry words to God were childish, unwarranted, and sinful, God was big enough to forgive me. Not having that bigness of heart and soul, it has been difficult to get my mind around such unconditional love, forgiveness and acceptance.

Tom's condition stabilized after several days, and he was moved to a step-down unit with more freedom. He could bathe with help, and wear his own pajamas. He could sit in a chair, have a telephone and a newspaper, and watch television. He was encouraged to walk. In the step down unit patients wore monitors day and night. Data from Tom's heart was signaled from the monitor via antennae in the ceilings of the rooms and halls to a constantly manned computer console in a room down the hall. It was a small step toward independence.

Tom, like many men, was adept at bottling up his emotions, a sometime sticking point in our relationship. He was not prepared when after the heart attack his emotions were near the surface and sometimes bubbled over as tears. Alone on a Sunday morning, he found himself not just weeping, but sobbing, as he sat in the chair in his room. To his horror, he could not seem to stop. Much to Tom's embarrassment one of our internists found him like this. Dr. James reassured Tom that being emotional after a heart attack was normal. He said that he thought the ancients might have been on to something when they identified the heart as the seat of human emotion. Tom had his emotions to deal with and I had my guilt. Neither of us shared much about his struggle with the other.

Still wearing his monitor twenty-four/seven, Tom improved slowly. He continued to have mild chest pain so he was placed on a regimen of nitrate therapy, and with nitroglycerin Tom's pain disappeared. He was able to walk more often and for further distances, and he passed his first post-heart-attack stress test.

Tom, as he felt better, chaffed at his restrictions-wearing the heart monitor was a nuisance; walking the same halls several times each day was boring. When I returned to the hospital for our next visit, Tom had been severely chastised for turning one too many corners and walking right off the monitor. Causing his heart beat to "straight line" on the computer had created a tense moment or two for everyone but Tom, who rounded the corner just in time to see frantic nurses running down the hall toward his room.

As Tom's health improved our communication improved, but there was much left unspoken and unacknowledged. We built a fragile bridge across the emotional chasm we had created while Tom was hospitalized and I was managing things at home and at work. I still filtered the answers I gave Tom when he questioned me about the business, leaving out any news that I deemed upsetting. Funny isn't it that I was doing to him the same thing he had done to me all those years, each of us acting with good intentions. He sensed that and resented it. I, on the other hand, resented that his post-heart attack status prevented me from seeking his input on business matters when I felt unsure of my own decisions. My feelings of resentment led to more feelings of guilt. We were each wounded and often silent. We did harm to our relationship and possibly to Tom's health in the name of caring.

For years, both before and after his first heart attack, Tom protected me by keeping any unfavorable business news from me. How did he do that when I was often at work in the same business? I wanted more to believe him than not. I enabled him. We both had come from families who owned and operated small businesses successfully over a period of many years. In both families I suppose business decisions were discussed and jointly made. I know they were in mine because as an only child I was often in the room for the discussions, my presence forgotten. Tom wanted more. As the business grew, he envisioned an ever bigger plant with more employees and a larger market. I wanted what Tom wanted. We both were caught up in the materialism rampant in an upwardly-mobile world. We were seeking the *American Dream* written in capital letters across the horizon in blinking neon lights in the last decades of the twentieth century.

The difficulty in writing this book is not in recalling all the bouts with heart disease and its attendant problems, procedures, and repairs. Tom and I agree that the difficulty is in being transparent. Acknowledging before the world the failures and foibles we each have is painful. Strangely, because I spent so many years denying that he had these particular ones, and sharing complicity in allowing them to continue, it is more difficult for me to mention Tom's failings than it is for me to catalogue my own. I thought I was being a good wife. Perhaps Tom is equally uncomfortable as he recognizes my shortcomings in print. I imagine us as being like Ebenezer Scrooge when he was confronted by the ugliness, and the rattling chains of Christmas Past. As uncomfortable and as unlike us as it is, we are both convinced that transparency is necessary if we are to paint a true picture of our lives. Perhaps our painful honesty will help others in similar situations to heal just as it has helped us. The healing has been a bonus we have discovered together as we have remembered and written; as we have prayed, praised God, and acknowledged His goodness and mercy to us.

4

Back In the Game

Tom became an entrepreneur by way of a career in research and then in management in a large manufacturing company after he had earned an advanced degree in physics. Tom held, through research he had done for the company, a couple of U.S. patents. He was an excellent, technically adept sales representative, and he had managed people and large projects. Tom had reached a plateau and needed a new challenge. More than that, Tom wanted a larger piece of the pie, and being his own boss sounded perfect.

In a borrowed space with an investment of less than a thousand dollars and the reluctant blessing of his employer, Tom and two other men started a part-time manufacturing company which produced custom made products complementary to the assembly-line pieces of the larger company where Tom still worked. The business thrived and moved to larger quarters. Eventually my husband left the larger factory to run his own small plant full time. One of the business' founding members left the new company; another remained as a mostly silent partner and sometime investor. As the oldest and the most experienced of the entrepreneurs, he coaxed Tom into visiting a respected banker, an old friend of his, who cautioned my husband about the difficulties of running a small business. Tom admits that he inwardly scoffed at the man's warnings against rapid growth as well as his other advice. As yet untested, Tom admits that he thought that for him, a scientist with an advanced degree and several years of experience in a large company, running a small business would be a piece of cake. Tom's energy

21

and enthusiasm overruled the misgivings of the more seasoned partner, and the factory moved into a new facility and hired more people.

I worked in the office answering the phones, assisting in the area of human resources and keeping the books. As a human resources advisor I shed some of my naiveté, learning that not all employees embraced my work ethic or my level of commitment to doing a good job. I disliked the confrontation that sometimes was necessary in holding someone accountable for doing a good job. Eventually I learned, as did Tom, that even when you tried your hardest to be a good and fair employer, you were not always perceived as such. I became, by default, the bookkeeper although I had no college business classes; I loathe math and had taken the minimum requirements. As a bookkeeper I had only three things going for me, a desire to help my husband, a passion for detail and organization, and patient lessons from a retired accountant who did oversee my work. When he told me accounts must balance to the penny, I became as diligent as the widow searching for her mite, though not with her spirituality. It was a red-letter day when I was introduced to adjusting entries.

These are the notions, realities, and attitudes we were dealing with when Tom came home from the hospital. We had a lot of baggage. Recuperative time from heart attacks in the 1980's was long, and for Tom it was tedious. Dr. Drew had told Tom and our family when we left the hospital that with advances in medicine and careful monitoring, he believed he could keep Tom ahead of the curve. He ventured that we might stay enough ahead of Tom's coronary artery disease to buy him five years before he would need surgery. We all heard the same message but Tom interpreted it to mean that he was cured; the heart attack had been a small bump in the road, and he had conquered it.

Once at home Tom quickly became bored with books, with television, and with computer games in spite of the fact that both cable television and personal computers had recently become available in our town. He changed channels incessantly as he lay in bed; he read sporadically; he played computer games on a computer loaned him by a friend. He even worked out a few manufacturing programs on the computer to use when he returned to the plant, but he chaffed at this enforced low-level activity.

I did not discuss work with Tom following the same pattern that I had while he had been hospitalized, afraid to do or to say anything that might cause my husband to worry. For the first time in our married lives I was the one to leave for the office each morning and he was the one staying home. Our inability to handle the situation almost wrecked our marriage.

In my efforts to protect Tom from any problems, I shut him out. He knew there were personnel problems, and that there was the potential of a forced buy-out by a stock-holding employee. Those problems had been brewing before his heart attack. He chose not to admit them to me or to bring them up in our conversation. Having been advised not to stress Tom, I was not going to bring up any of the problems. Tom became jealous of the time I spent away from him. He felt useless. I felt exhausted and out of my depth. During this time when we were both so fragile and vulnerable, a loved and trusted person said that perhaps the stress leading to Tom's heart attack was created by the secrets he was keeping from me. There was likely some truth in those words, but the inference was that there might be another woman in Tom's life. I knew Tom was not immune to feminine beauty when he saw it, but the one sure thing that had always turned his head came with wings and a propeller. If it was not an airplane, I was reasonably confident that Tom was not interested. He remained the one man in my life and I, the one woman in his. Tom and I had issues we needed to face, but infidelity was not one of them. The attempt to plant that seed of doubt, especially by someone close to us, was another secret I had to keep, and it hurt me deeply.

Tom had the first of what must be a record number of heart catheterizations-thirty-just three weeks after being discharged from the hospital. Having passed that hurdle, Tom returned to work at the factory where things really had not changed much. All the crises and frustrations that attend the rapid growth of a small company were still there, and Tom maintained control of it all, partly of necessity, but largely because that is the way he wanted it. I wish we could say that with what we had experienced during Tom's first bout with heart disease we learned and we made changes in our work-related habits, but in retrospect we did not-we only thought we did.

Tom continued to believe that he functioned best under stress; he continued to be less than forthcoming about some business issues, and I continued to enable that habit. Tom, pronouncing himself *cured,* though never a sedentary person, found time only sporadically for aerobic exercise. He smoked the occasional cigar, not inhaling made it okay long before that phrase became part of our political pop culture. I did change cooking habits, hiding the salt shaker, and the frying pan, and serving desserts far less often. My attempts to enforce a healthy diet were not altogether successful. There were often candy wrappers and empty cashew packages stuffed under the car seat or in the pocket of the car door.

Not much had really changed. I realized how apt Dr. John's description of Tom had been shortly after the heart attack. He had called Tom a *duck*--calm on the surface and paddling like hell underneath. It should have been no surprise when two and a half years after that first myocardial infarction Tom became symptomatic. Exertion made him short of breath and he was having chest pain. Tom was scheduled for a second heart cath. We had failed an important lesson in accountability. Tom largely ignored the need to make changes in his lifestyle. Diet, lack of exercise, and stress-always stress-were working against him. I pleaded and cajoled about diet and exercise, but I did not confront Tom about things in, the runaway growth of the business that I knew were stressors. He still chose not to be forthcoming and I, even though I sensed most of the problems, still chose not to make him acknowledge that I knew about them.

A heart catheterization is an invasive procedure and not without risk. The needle, guide wire, and catheter are inserted by a cardiologist into the femoral artery in the groin. They are snaked upward into the heart where, using a dye for contrast, pictures called angiograms are taken of the heart to show any abnormalities in the shape and contour of the vessels in the heart. The cardiologist can also use this tool to check pressures in the heart's pumping system, and to determine if its valves are functioning properly. It is a great tool for assessing the state of the heart. When the procedure is complete the catheter is withdrawn through the artery in the groin, and pressure is applied to the entry wound. At this early stage of Tom's heart disease, the regimen required the patient to lie flat of his back with no pillow and no movement for at least eight hours until the entry site had clotted sufficiently to prevent bleeding. Tom's heart catheterization showed right coronary artery lesions ranging from seventy to ninety percent. His left coronary artery now exhibited lesser lesions. The disease had progressed. Overall the heart had more blockage than it had previously shown. This catheterization also showed us an amazing development. The portion of Tom's heart damaged by the infarction two and a half years previous had developed something called a Kugel's artery. This tiny vessel sometimes develops where a larger artery has been blocked or severely damaged. It was giving a portion of that heart muscle that we had expected to be dead, just enough blood supply to keep it alive. It is as if God has provided a fail-safe system in our bodies. Tom was released from the hospital with some changes in his medication, and the addition of a nitroglycerin patch he was to wear to dilate the vessels that were becoming more blocked. He was admonished to get better control of his diabetes.

People's lives rarely have just one thin thread of a story; instead, they are tapestries woven of multiple joys, sorrows, triumphs, and things we wish we had done better. Our experiences were no different. Our children were growing up and making us proud of their accomplishments. One was accepted to a prestigious university; the other, still in high school, was exhibiting talents in the arts. I had major surgery. Our parents aged; one became ill. Our lives were quite ordinary. The manufacturing plant continued to grow. We became involved in building material for the booming oil and gas market in the Permian Basin of West Texas. Tom spent a good bit of time there. He enjoyed the people, the excitement of the boom, and the wide open vistas. Like a lot of other folks in the eighties we were chasing the good life as defined by bigger homes, vacation homes, boats-all the good stuff. We were becoming overextended emotionally, physically, and economically, but we did not acknowledge it. We were caught up in acquiring things, and a relationship with our Creator was not our top priority. It was not the things we wanted or the things we acquired that were wrong; it was the place in our hearts that we gave to those things that undermined our foundation. Tom was still that duck paddling furiously. I was silent although I was aware that Tom was pushing the outer limits of the amount of stress we could handle. I did not want to admit that I saw chinks in his armor and I did not want to be accused of nagging. Confrontation-I avoided it. Tom and I were not selfish. We gave time, money, and effort to good causes. We felt a certain amount of civic responsibility, and we were involved in groups to help our community. We volunteered in our children's schools. We attended church on a regular basis, teaching, and serving on committees. We were doing so many things right but we continued to assume total control of our lives, running to God most often when we wanted Him to see things our way. In our effort to control, we almost lost everything, even Tom's life.

Not yet fifty years old, Tom was back in the hospital for his third heart catheterization five years and seven days after his initial heart attack. The business was flourishing with one branch in our hometown and another in the oil fields of West Texas. Tom was still attempting to wear all the hats-CEO, manager, head of research and development, and technical service. He appeared to be juggling all the duties well, but the stress was taking its toll. In October when business in the Permian Basin hit a slump, the tension in the office and at home was tangible. Tom was traveling regularly from Arkansas to West Texas, and on one of his trips he developed pain in his jaw, a sometime warning of impending heart problems.

Dr. Drew ordered a treadmill test which was abnormal, indicating a progression of Tom's coronary artery disease. A third catheterization was ordered because it was the most reliable tool for seeing what was going on in my husband's heart. There was little change to the left side of the organ, but on the right side Tom now had two ninety percent lesions and a near total blockage in the right coronary artery. This cath was notable not only for the increased blockage, but also because it was the only catheterization ever done through one of Tom's brachial arteries. The cardiologist went in through Tom's right arm. This arteriogram was also the first to show a drop in the ejection fraction of Tom's heart. The ejection fraction measures the heart's pumping efficiency. The ability of Tom's heart to pump was not badly compromised and was still within a range considered normal, but it had fallen five percent in two years, foreshadowing problems we would encounter later. Tom left the hospital on five medications with plans to add a sixth, an anticoagulant to reduce the load on his damaged heart, as soon as we returned from a trip we had planned to visit our son on his college campus.

Why did Tom leave each heart-related incident believing he was cured? I do not know. Perhaps he really did not believe that and was just whistling in the dark. Perhaps he was simply putting on a brave front although I do not believe that is true. We all view events through our own peculiar lenses. Tom was, and is still, a very positive person with a tremendous capacity to view life as the glass half full. It is this trait, second only to God's grace, which has kept him going. It is also the trait that has, at times, blinded him to reality. I, less of an optimist, continued to hide my feelings and my fears. I felt, rightly or wrongly, that I was pushed to be the strong oak when I longed to be a weeping willow. Reading back through my journals I find that I sounded incredibly needy with a weak and wavering faith. Tom and I were often at odds over his health issues; I hovered and he resisted. He had his running shoes on and was racing through life while I was waiting for the other shoe to fall. I had hit a new low one difficult spring day when I wrote melodramatically in a journal.

When did Sandra die I wonder.
When did her soul flee?
When did this drudge fill her shell
I wonder.

Bereft of laughter and joy,
When did Sandra die I wonder.
And what is left of me?

Melodramatic? Admittedly. Heartfelt? Probably. Afraid to trust God completely, I was overwhelmed a great deal of the time, if not publicly, then certainly in the privacy of my journal and in the long nights I lay awake with all the *what-ifs* playing themselves out in my mind.

In the early eighties, a cousin of mine received a heart transplant after a virus attacked his heart causing cardiomyopathy. Until then we had known no one who had received a heart transplant. I signed a donor card. In those days a donor carried a card, and a sticker was placed on the windshield of his car indicating his intentions. The windshield sticker was quite a source of concern for our young daughter. Not understanding the donor process, she was unwilling to sit on that side of the car until I assured her that neither she nor I would lose our hearts as long as we had need of them. It is a child's view of things, but I mention it in order to say that world-wide many people, through fear or ignorance, choose not to sign donor cards. God bless those families who, out of their own sorrow, give the gift of life.

In the summer of 1986, our still expanding company got a contract from an oil company to build some large parts that were to be completed in Brownsville, Texas and floated to Dubai. Tom, elated, loved the challenge. Frightened because he continued to take on more responsibility and more stress, I was less enthusiastic but silent about his latest project. I sensed that Tom was worse. He was short of breath; he became irritable more easily, indicators I was learning to view as flashing yellow caution lights. At his regularly scheduled appointment with Dr. Drew we heard the familiar mantra; Tom was to monitor his diabetes more closely; he was to add another pill to those he was already swallowing, and he was to return in early February for another check-up. The cardiologist had not told my husband, as I had hoped he would, that Tom had to make drastic changes in his life style. I was disappointed. Tom was pleased to hear, through whatever filter he used, that he was fine to go as on before. I felt as if the sword of Damocles was hanging by a single thread over our heads. We had one child in university a thousand miles away, one in the third year of high school, and a couple of parents nearby who had some health issues of their own, and my husband refused to see his heart problems as a progressive disease. Five days after that appointment, Tom was on a plane to Brownsville, Texas to check the Dubai project.

That January Tom made a final trip to the Port of Brownsville to inspect the Dubai job before it was floated to the Persian Gulf. The inspection required that Tom climb stairs and ladders equal to the height of a five story building; with this exertion his angina returned and worsened. His color was bad, and he had difficulty breathing. The two factory workers Tom had taken along from our plant to help with the inspection were frightened by my husband's obvious pain and distress. They insisted that he should go home. That they prevailed is a sure indicator that Tom felt worse than he would acknowledge. He drove himself to the nearest airport in Harlingen, Texas, and caught the first available flight home. Tom had been home for just a few moments when he admitted the difficulty and pain he had experienced while climbing the ladders. I realized that Tom was frightened when he called Dr. Drew without objecting. That afternoon Tom underwent his fourth heart catheterization. Following the cath procedure Dr. Drew came to the waiting room to talk with our family and some of our friends. When you are an only child as I am, close friends become the sisters and brothers you never had. Dr. Drew mapped Tom's heart for us explaining that his disease had progressed to the point that my husband needed a quadruple by-pass. Tom was not awake from the procedure and did not yet know what lay ahead; that he was scheduled for surgery the next morning, February 19, 1987. Dr. Drew said he would explain things to Tom as soon as he awoke. Before going to make arrangements for a surgeon for Tom, and to secure a room in the coronary care unit where my husband would spend the night, the doctor also suggested that I should try to reach our son, Tad, to tell him to fly home immediately from the East Coast where he was in college. I tried without success to reach Tad. When Dr. Drew came back by the waiting room and heard that I had exhausted all our change and most of my calm without talking to Tad, he called his office staff telling them to book our son's flight and to call him until they reached him. Frazzled as I was, this kindness brought tears to my eyes. As he turned to leave, the doctor told my mother-in-law and me that Tom was awake, and that we could see him; what Dr. Drew did not say was that he had not yet explained to Tom that he would be staying in the hospital to have surgery the following morning. My mother-in-law and I rushed into the room with damp eyes and fixed smiles telling Tom that he was not to worry. We looked like harbingers of doom. Tom says that one look at us coupled with the dread *don't worry* phrase convinced him we had come to tell him he was dying. He vows that our demeanor made it much easier to hear that he was *only* to have quadruple by-pass surgery the following morning. Tom was relieved we had not come to bury him.

Our dear friend, James, brought Tad from the airport to the hospital late that afternoon. Tom was moved to CCU and met his surgeon. Leigh came to the hospital after school although I do not recall how or with whom. Perhaps I trusted her as I had her brother five years earlier to drive herself there. With Tom once again in CCU we were back to strictly regulated visiting hours. The children and I went home to take care of all the loose ends caused by this unexpected turn of events, and to prepare for the wait we would face tomorrow while Tom was in surgery. While at home I called one of the three teaching pastors at our church, told him the situation, and asked for his prayers, and those of the congregation. Bill prayed right then as I held the phone to my ear. I had never experienced phone prayer, and I was both comforted and surprised. God was doing as He promises and providing for my needs at the time those needs arose.

Back at the hospital Tom's mind was awhirl with all that had transpired. He even began to think that maybe his *warranty* was running out. The surgeon came by Tom's room before I got back to CCU. His description of the surgery was precise; I was sorry that I had not heard it. Tom and I visited our allotted time without being able to say all that was in our hearts and minds; our conversation was stilted. As visiting hours were ending Pastor Bill, who had prayed on the telephone with me came to Tom's room. He brought with him Robert, the lead pastor, whom we barely knew. We gratefully accepted Robert's offer to pray for us. Pastor Robert did pray for Tom and *Sarah*, but I was sure that God knew my name even if Robert didn't, and this slip of the tongue has provided us all with many a smile in the years since. In spite of being closeted again in a small, windowless space Tom says he felt calmed and uplifted after the prayers. The apprehension Tom had felt was replaced with the realization, at least for a while, that he was in the hands of our Creator.

I wasn't allowed to stay in the room with Tom so I drove home planning to be at the hospital early the next morning. The children and I wanted to see Tom before he was taken to the surgery suite. That night Tom remembers that the cardiologist and the anesthesiologist visited him. A male nurse Tom remembers as one of the kindest health professionals he encountered in what became a large cast of such folks, shaved his chest, belly, and legs in preparation for the surgery. When he left, Tom was at peace and able to sleep.

Tad, Leigh, and I returned in the pre-dawn light to Tom's room in the CCU. He was awake, and after taking the prescribed happy pill, he was almost jovial as an IV was started to help him relax and become sleepy. Part of the light-heartedness was for our benefit, I think, and hard as we tried to match his mood our smiles were shaky. Have you ever considered how difficult it is to say anything important at such a time? Your heart and mind are full of love, and, fear, and memories that resist being formed into a coherent sentence.

The attendant came to move Tom, who was now groggy, to the O.R. holding area. The children and I were allowed to come along. Tom, who has been a pilot since he was fourteen, spread his arms widely as he lay on the moving gurney. Tom was *flying*. When he *landed* the four of us joined hands and prayed. We kissed him goodbye, and he was gone through the double doors into the OR and someone else's hands. You can believe in a surgeon's proficiency, his staff's competence, and even that God is in charge, but in the second that those surgery suite doors close there is a finality that sends your heart to your toes and a lump to your throat.

5

The Cabbage

Tom's coronary artery disease and unstable angina had placed him face up on an operating table. Cold, stripped naked, and supine, he gratefully accepted the warm blanket someone wrapped around him. He could hear chit chat among the technicians and nurses, and then nothing. Tom's left leg was prepped from the groin to below the knee in order to recover his greater saphenous vein for the needed grafts, those Coronary Artery Bypass Grafts familiarly called CABG's or *cabbages*. The vein, once removed from Tom's leg, was rinsed and prepared for use. The leg wound was closed. The operating team then turned their attention to Tom's chest. Using a saw the surgeon cracked the sternum and began carefully dissecting to expose the heart with its great vessels or arteries. He attached Tom's heart to the by-pass machine in order to maintain its function. Next he dropped Tom's body temperature to about twenty eight degrees centigrade. The surgeon and his team bathed the sac around Tom's heart, the pericardium, in an iced saline solution. They clamped the aorta and chose the sites for the bypass grafts. In Tom's case, areas on the first and second posterior descending branches of the right coronary artery were prepared. Two additional grafts were constructed for Tom's heart. When all the grafts were in place the clamps were released. Tom's surgeon ascertained that the grafts were successful and not leaking. The team began the process of weaning Tom from the cardiopulmonary bypass machine and allowing circulation through the patched arteries to feed his heart. The surgeon closed the wound in Tom's chest.

After spending some time in the recovery room, Tom was wheeled back to the intensive coronary care unit, pale, full of tubes, and still heavily anesthetized. He was unaware of the team that had labored to heal him or of the family and friends waiting and praying. When I first glimpsed Tom his face was puffy and pale; his eyes were swollen and shut; his lips were swollen. There seemed to be tubes everywhere in every orifice, and a respirator was doing his breathing. The surgeon told Tad, Leigh, and me that Tom had come through the operation well, and that he was doing fine. We had to accept those words on faith since appearances did not lead us to that conclusion. We each kissed Tom, or tried to get close enough through all of his life support machinery to kiss him, and we returned to the waiting room. As Tom began his return from the abyss of unconsciousness, he heard voices but he could not open his eyes. He wondered if the voices were his introduction to heaven. He was aware of a bright light focused on his eyelids. At that instant he heard a voice inquire if anyone had ordered pizza-he was pretty sure he was still earthbound. There were nurses at the foot of his bed and one beside him who urged him to take a deep breath. Tom was surprised to find that he could do that. When he inhaled, the attendant yanked the ventilator tube from his mouth, and Tom was breathing on his own. Seven days later my husband was released from the hospital and instructed to return to the cardiologist's office in three weeks for a treadmill test. He was told not to drive for six weeks or until his sternum healed.

Life returned to what passed for normal. Our son went back east to complete his junior year of college, and our daughter returned to her junior year in high school. Although we did not talk about it the children and I, and, I think, Tom's parents and mine, realized that we would most likely face more bouts with Tom's coronary artery disease. Tom never allowed that thought to gain purchase in his mind. Once more he left the hospital *cured*. My husband, still hugging the heart-shaped pillow the nurse had given to him to hold when he coughed, held staff meetings in our dining room within days of his release from the hospital. Recovery time after Tom's first surgery was shorter by far than his recovery had been after his heart attack.

Tom was fascinated by the mechanical workings of the heart and its vessels. He asked tons of questions about the procedures that were to be done to him. The science of the pressures and flows of the circulatory system and the problems encountered when there were blockages intrigued him. He found similarities to the piping systems he designed and repaired for industry. In later years when he faced more surgeries he would badger Tad into bringing his medical texts to the hospital so they could pour over the heart-related chapters before Tom was taken to surgery. I never shared his enthusiasm for these *learning opportunities*.

From the onset of Tom's heart problems we did rely on faith though that reliance was often weak and incomplete. With each new twist and turn we were challenged to go deeper in our relationship with the Lord. Sometimes we made good progress along that road, and at times we did not. Once in a while well-meaning but misinformed believers threw roadblocks in our path. After Tom's surgery I sensed that something was eating at our daughter's faith and heart. Because she knew how burdened I was with business, home, and an incapacitated husband, she was reluctant to share with me that a youth-group friend had told her that if she had only prayed harder her father would not have required surgery. As Leigh and I talked about sharing incomplete and immature concepts, even in good faith, we were able to work through her feelings that she was somehow responsible for her dad's poor health. In our one step forward, two steps back fashion; our family progressed in our faith journey. Tom's first Sunday back in church after his surgery the pastor asked the congregation, as he sometimes does, to share concerns and praises. Rising, Tom took the microphone and thanked God for His grace, and he thanked the congregation for their prayers and kindness. I was surprised by such uncharacteristic openness on my husband's part, but I suspect God and His angels cheered. Trembling from the exertion of standing, and from emotion, Tom dropped to his seat. He had opened the door a little wider to the Father who will not come into our hearts unbidden. I would like to say that our faith, individually and as a family, followed a smooth and uncluttered path from that moment on, but that would be a lie. We, inconsistent and often weak, followed as the country song says *a broken road*.

Upon his six-week examination by the surgeon, Tom was pronounced healing well and fit to drive. The post-op visit to Dr. Drew was not as pleasant. The cardiologist, as he had after Tom's heart attack, said that if my husband was a compliant patient, taking medicines as prescribed, exercising regularly, and following his diet, they could probably buy him five years before further intervention was necessary. Five years! That was nothing. Tom wanted a lifetime-thirty, even forty years. Although he was reasonably compliant in diet and exercise, and very good about his prescriptions, Tom kept upping the ante in his gamble with stress. Back at work, he hit the ground running. Refusing to admit that the business had more challenges than any one person could meet; he kept juggling all the balls and wearing all the hats.

Just over a month after Tom was released from the hospital we, with our daughter, were on the beaches of the Florida panhandle for Spring Break. Tom self-consciously sported his still pink, mid-chest scar. Months rolled by. Our son graduated college and started medical school. Our daughter graduated high school and started college in another state. We gave the appearance of managing the business and our lives reasonably well. In truth the stress increased incrementally, generated by all the ups and downs of entrepreneurship, by Tom's efforts to hide any bad news from me, and by my refusal to confront him when I knew that was what he was doing. Our spiritual growth remained an on again, off again thing. Our communication skills with each other suffered from a lack of transparency on both our parts. We were not always kind to each other but we persevered, putting a good face on things as people do. As we chased material gain and pride of place we cheated no one; we intentionally hurt no one, except each other. We went to church, we loved our families, and we supported the right civic organizations. We ran hard to get it all covered, and the more we ran, the harder we needed to run to keep everything going physically, economically, and socially. Emotionally and spiritually we might not have been bankrupt, but our ledgers were full of red ink.

6

Revisiting the Cabbage Patch

The cardiologist must have had a crystal ball because in five years and three months Tom's coronary artery bypass grafts needed patching. Dr. Drew's routine examination of Tom indicated that he needed another arteriogram. The physician who had done Tom's original surgery had retired, so four days after the arteriogram, June 8, 1992; Dr. Michael became Tom's cardiac surgeon and successfully completed five by-pass grafts on his heart. Three of the five were re-dos of those grafts made in Tom's first heart surgery. One of the old grafts to Tom's right coronary artery had one hundred percent blockage. There was also blockage in my husband's left anterior descending artery, making both sides of his heart now subject to this progressive disease. Dr. Michael used more of Tom's saphenous veins as well as his mammary artery to build the grafts he needed. We were excited about the use of the mammary because we had read that those grafts made of arteries frequently lasted longer than those made of veins. Eight days after a recovery that is called *unremarkable* in physicians' notes, Tom was home again. He had a little fluid in the left chest cavity but no signs of pneumonia. It was noted that his heart was slightly enlarged; a forerunner of heart failure, but its size was not yet beyond normal limits. Reading the notes of both the surgeon and the cardiologist, Tom and I are again struck by what skillful physicians they are, and how blessed we have been to have them as his doctors. There is no way to overestimate the importance of our growing relationship with these two men. Their God-given knowledge and skills kept Tom alive.

We would have been bereft without them and without the unflagging support of family and friends. It is our firm belief that God placed each of these persons in our lives so that their strengths would shore up our weaknesses.

In recalling all the kindnesses we were shown and the love we were freely given, Tom and I fear leaving someone out, and we do not want to do that. There are instances which, though they may seem insignificant to the others involved, stand boldly in our memories. Some occurred after this surgery, some earlier or later in our journey. We are thankful for them all. After Tom's heart attack I remember driving to the home of a childhood friend and sitting in her kitchen crying, which she allowed me to do. With two children and a recuperating husband at home I did not have the luxury of opening those floodgates in my own house. We remember church friends who prayed, sent cards and brought meals. We were blessed with family, especially our parents, who pitched in to take up the slack wherever possible. With each surgery so many of our friends and family came to sit with us that I think the hospital hostesses were overwhelmed. Each hospitalization the Fiser contingent looked a little like a small convention. People came and went; they prayed, held our hands, and hugged us as we all waited. The time waiting always seemed long, and with each surgery it was longer; the surgery was more risky. I think there was a communal sigh of relief every time Dr. Michael appeared to tell us that an operation on Tom's heart had been a successful one.

Some memories make us smile such as the story of Tom's *fourth sister.* He has only three, but a long-time friend outsmarted hospital rules by becoming a relative and getting into the ICU to see my husband shortly after more than one surgery. Perhaps it would take another only child, as a toddler our daughter had called it *lonely child,* and that was true, to understand how much this great wave of visible support meant to me. Without it I would have retreated into a small dark cave with nothing but my fears. God provided these friends and prayer warriors to lift us up and they each blessed us in their own special way. There were the unexpected moments, shocking at the time, which we look back on with laughter. After Tom's heart attack or his first surgery, we cannot recall which, our ski boat needed to be winterized. I didn't know how to do it so a neighbor and his son were helping Tad with that chore as the boat sat in our driveway. From next door another neighbor, a gregarious New Englander of Italian descent, bounded out his back door announcing without preamble that if Tom *didn't make it,* he would sure like to buy the boat. We were speechless.

To prove that his heart was in the right place even if his foot was in his mouth, our Italian neighbor cooked Tom a homecoming dinner of the best veal Marsala we have ever eaten. I remember when our son's fraternity brothers, one Jewish and one Muslim, told Tad that they were praying for his father. I remember our daughter's best friends in high school being there for her at the hospital and at home. I remember later the college friend whose home was in Memphis who frequently made the drive to Little Rock to offer Leigh her support. I remember the medical school classmate of our son's who sat late at night in the darkened waiting room and rubbed my swollen feet. There was the friend and neighbor who in those pre-cell phone days emptied his pockets of quarters each time he visited the hospital to be certain that I always had change for the pay phone. There were two special women who completed an antique quilt begun by my great grandmother and presented it to me one Christmas just to cheer me. I remember delicious meals, and shared cleaning ladies, and more kindnesses than I could ever enumerate or repay.

After Tom's second surgery his best friend, one of the founding members of a large and successful Arkansas company, said that he wanted to help run our business. Having retired early perhaps James was bored, but I think that mostly he saw a need that he could meet. James became our mentor, our hard-headed business associate, and our stickler for details. He referred to himself as *the wart*. He was our confidant, and closer to us both than a brother. He and his wife were our longtime friends. We were with them the weekend Tom gave up cigarettes and James couldn't. He tried and failed several times over the years. If ever there was an argument for tobacco as an addiction, he was it.

Our physicians were both supremely professional, but in time we began to look on them as not only our doctors, but as our friends. Tad did an elective rotation with one of them during his third year of medical school. Upon learning that she shared a love for Carolina beach music with our cardiologist, Leigh made him a tape of it for listening to in the cath lab. Dr. Drew and Dr. Michael practice the art as well as the science of medicine. We count our relationship with them as a tremendous blessing.

1993 proved to be eventful. Tom and I made our dream trip in late March to the British Isles. We did all the planning ourselves and made the arrangements. When we landed at Heathrow we rented a car and drove, for us Americans, on the wrong side of the road through England, Ireland, Scotland, and Wales. It was a magical time. We cannot regret it though in retrospect, for reasons both economic and physical, we should probably have stayed at home. That spring we learned that both of our children were engaged, and that both would be married before the year was out.

1995 was the year Tom's heart lost its ability to go five years between surgeries. By June 7, increasing shortness of breath and fatigue put him back in the hospital for heart catheterization number six-that seemed like such a lot of them. Little did we know that the number of catheterizations would more than quadruple in the coming years. The procedure revealed that Tom's right coronary artery was again occluded, the anterior descending vessel was seventy percent blocked, and the proximal portion of the circumflex was one hundred percent blocked. The biggest disappointment was that the internal mammary artery bypass graft, which Dr. Michael had described after the second surgery as *a huge honker*, was one hundred percent blocked. Our physicians, our family and, most assuredly, the patient were dismayed at the increasingly rapid progression of the disease.

Those times as we stumbled from surgery to surgery were difficult. We were riding an emotional roller coaster. If we had not been able to find humor in our situation sometimes, I do not think we would have survived. I think God gave us this ability to laugh at ourselves in the midst of what could well become a tragic situation. Our laughter was to us what a steam valve is to a pressure cooker; it kept us from exploding. On one such occasion Tom's best friend stopped by the hospital to visit the night before a surgery. He walked into the room to find Tom and Tad with medical texts spread on the bed, and the two of them deep in a discussion of the heart's sinuses and angioplasty. Our friend's face registered increasing discomfort and incredulity as he listened to father and son. Thinking of the only sinuses he was familiar with, he asked if the doctor would really guide the catheter to Tom's heart through his nose. I do not think he was at all reassured when they explained that the sinuses were in the heart but that the catheter came up from the groin. Through the nose or through the groin, each seemed to James to be a long road to the heart. We sometimes forgot that our exposure to medical terminology, at least that referring to the heart, exceeded the norm.

Even at the darkest times it was sometimes a moment of unintentional humor that kept us going. After Tom's second surgery our ten-year-old nephew, who was pretty fond of his Uncle Tom, crept stealthily from the CVICU waiting room down a long hall toward the intensive care unit. Exhausted and absorbed in our own thoughts, we adults didn't realize Justin was missing until Dr. Michael collared him and deposited him back in the waiting room. Justin was embarrassed, and angry, and still worried about this uncle he could not visit. He also knew that his mother was not happy with him and that there were words and attitudes that she would not tolerate from him. Justin sat red-faced and scowling until a friend of ours, a teacher accustomed to ten-year-old boys, asked if he was angry. Justin answered that yes he was. Our friend asked Justin to tell her just how angry he felt. Justin looked at his mother, and turning to Linda asked if she knew where the devil lived because *that* was how mad he was. We successfully (for the most part) hid our smiles and the story lives on in family lore.

I have written a lot about Tom's refusal to recognize that what he had was a progressive disease. That was still true, at least to outward appearances. We had, though, long since changed our eating habits for the healthier. Tom was faithful to his medication schedule. Exercise was still sporadic but he remained active. Tobacco use was a distant memory, even the cigars he had once enjoyed on rare occasions. Alcohol intake was the rare glass of wine or Scotch. On the other hand business related stress continued to increase as Tom delegated too little and took on too much. Tom's mild diabetes was never under great control even though we were able to manage it with oral medication rather than insulin injections. Tom and I believe that we underestimated the role of diabetes in his disease, but we believe that above all other factors, stress was the culprit attacking his heart.

During catheterization six my husband experienced ventricular tachycardia and required cardioversion. In layman's terms, they used the paddles on him. Did he flat line? I do not know, thank God. The cardiologist's report states only the facts and that there were no consequences noted. Ever the inquisitive scientist, Tom liked watching the display of his heart and its vessels on the screen as Dr. Drew catheterized his heart. During number six Tom remembers tracking the fluorescence on the monitor as the dye coursed through the tentacles of his circulatory system. One moment he was watching the monitor, and in the next his vision went black, and Dr. Drew was standing over him ordering him, in an uncharacteristically loud voice, not to do that again. Tom's arteries were once more blocked. He was discharged with orders to restrict his activity and to return in about a week for surgery.

7

Re-Doing the Re-Dos

Eleven days shy of our thirty-third wedding anniversary Tom underwent his third surgery for coronary artery disease. Operative reports are a terse statement of fact. This one reads that the surgery was a "re-do, re-do coronary artery by-pass grafting x 5 with separate saphenous vein grafts" to each of the five sites. Dr. Michael, once again our surgeon, noted that two of the grafts were "T'd due to paucity of vein;" three surgeries and fourteen grafts, counting originals and re-dos, use up a lot of resources. It was a difficult surgery by any measure because the surgeon was dealing with adhesions and scar tissue from all the previous chest crackings. It is remarkable that once again Tom's recovery was noted to be *unremarkable.* I suppose this is an apt description in the sense that Tom had no problems coming off the ventilator and breathing on his own; that he had no difficulties with the incisions in his legs or with his legs swelling. To me, however, each successful surgery seemed not only remarkable, but a miracle allowing our children and me more time with the man we loved.

One of the things I have failed to mention thus far is that prior to being diagnosed with heart disease, Tom had developed an allergy to aspirin; it caused his throat to swell and most likely would have sent him into anaphylactic shock. Using aspirin as a blood thinner, as is so often done prophylactically, was not an option for him. He required a prescription drug, one of the eight medications he was taking when he left the hospital. The discharge summary noted that his blood pressure was acceptable; his diabetes was under reasonable control for one who had just had surgery, and his overall heart size was judged to be in the upper limits of normal. We took him home with instructions to see the surgeon for a post-op visit in four weeks and the cardiologist in six.

It was about this time that Tom became closer friends with a man approximately the same age and with many heart problems similar to his own. They had met through membership in a civic club to which they both belonged. There were differences in their disease and differences in their attitudes toward the coronary artery disease that plagued them both. Tom's friend watched his diet carefully; Tom was content to let me plan his diet. The other fellow exercised religiously and maintained an ideal weight. Tom still exercised sporadically and his weight was a little high. Both men were small business owners facing a fair amount of stress in their jobs. Both were married and the fathers of two children. They saw the same cardiologist. Often they used lunches at their club as a time to compare notes and to encourage each other in their fight against coronary artery disease. The friend had an air of concern about his condition while Tom still put any frightening possibilities that might lie ahead in some sort of box and closed the lid. Tom's attitude remained one of his greatest strengths as well as his Achilles heel. It certainly frustrated me most of the time.

One day and fourteen months after Tom's third surgery Dr. Drew conducted another arteriogram on my husband because of the angina he was experiencing. The procedure showed blockages ranging from twenty to one hundred percent in various vessels. The ejection fraction of the heart was still good at fifty percent, meaning that the muscle was strong enough to pump adequately. The blockages were, for the most part, on the left side of Tom's heart with the right side remaining open allowing a normal right ventricular function. After consultation with the surgeon, the cardiologist chose to treat Tom medically with no further invasive procedures at that time. Tom had undergone his third coronary artery bypass grafting a scant year earlier. A relatively young man, my husband was running out of vessels to be used in grafts-those remaining needed to be conserved. As far as I have been able to learn, there had been at that time no successful grafts from donors or any made from synthetic materials.

In another sixteen months Tom presented to his cardiologist with chest pain. His stress echocardiogram was abnormal. He was again hospitalized for heart catheterization during which a stent was placed in his left anterior descending bypass. The hospital team monitored him for forty eight hours. When they saw that he was doing well, he was released. In another forty eight hours he was back at the plant working. We thought an easier fix had been found for Tom. Implanting a stent was still an invasive procedure, but it certainly did not present the risk involved in cracking the chest for full blown heart bypass surgery. Both Tom and Dr. Drew had high hopes for the stent, then a relatively new development in the treatment of clogged arteries. In a matter of months those hopes were dashed when the stent in Tom's artery occluded.

It was obvious to all of us that Tom had lost the five years between surgeries that Dr. Drew had talked about, the magic number for hopefully keeping my husband on the cutting edge of medical knowledge and technology in the battle with his progressive coronary artery disease. Families, I think, adapt to such situations by making the most of every moment they are together, or at least ours did. The holidays that had always been important family times became more so. At Christmas our out-of-state children and our three precious grandchildren came home for an extended visit. We enjoyed the church services celebrating the birth of our Lord and Savior, especially the children's service where each of the toddlers got to hang an ornament on the congregational tree. We gathered in the kitchen to make apple Santas just as I had done as a child. We baked and iced a birthday cake for the baby Jesus-at least some of the icing went on the cake; a good deal of it went on little hands and faces, and our oldest granddaughter who was only three, solemnly iced the feet of the eleven month old sitting on the counter by the cake. We celebrated the Christ child's birthday with gusto. All our family times, whether around the tree, around the pool, or somewhere else were made more special by our unspoken awareness that each time might be the last. This is, at least, the way that our children and I felt. Tom would have no part of such thoughts so our unspoken fear became the elephant in the room. Perhaps Tom thought if he acknowledged the elephant it might trample him. Tom and I each had idiosyncrasies we developed dealing with his disease. If his was to refuse to acknowledge its presence most of the time, then mine was to quit sleeping with my head on his chest. In all of our married years I had at least started the night snuggled close to him with my head on his chest. I developed what I suppose could rightfully be called a phobia about having my ear over his heart and hearing its beat as I fell asleep. What if it stopped? In my mind, like the tell-tale heart in Poe's story, Tom's heart grew louder and louder as I lay with my head pressed against his chest, and I could not sleep for fear that it would stop. I made all sorts of excuses for my change in sleeping habits, and Tom never pressed me for the truth.

My husband entered the hospital in April 1998, with chest pain radiating down his left arm. He had an emergency heart catheterization. The hospital records do not number his catheterizations, but I think the count at this point was approaching double digits. The arteriography picture was not pretty; it showed more blockage and greater progression of the disease. There were four areas of my husband's heart with occlusions ranging from thirty to ninety-five percent. The cardiologist, as he always did to help explain Tom's situation, drew a heart map. The picture it presented was worth a thousand words-none of them encouraging.

8

Do We Have a Fourth?

In the months prior to his fourth surgery Tom's health and stamina declined. We moved his office from the manufacturing plant, several miles away, to our guest house, which at different times previously, had served as the post-college home of each of our children. For many reasons this was not a perfect situation; a manager needs to be on site every day. The little house sat about a football field's distance down a steep hill from our home with a swimming pool between the two. That hill became ever more difficult for Tom to navigate, but neither of us wanted the office physically in our home. We had tried that in the past and given Tom's personality, his work days grew longer in direct proportion to the proximity of his office. I worked with Tom as much as possible tending to secretarial duties and other things I could do in this home office. Much of my time, however, was taken caring for an elderly aunt and uncle, childless and in poor health. They were more like grandparents to me than aunt and uncle; I was glad to be able to help care for them.

Tom's best friend, James, continued as advisor and liaison to the manufacturing plant. Most days he joined us in the guest house we had converted to office space. James still smoked, unable to break the habit in spite of all his attempts, but his cigarette breaks were always outside the office away from Tom and me. James had his annual physical and told us that he had been pronounced fit. He was making plans to take Janet on an extended vacation out of the country. When Tom and I learned just days later that Tom would be facing a fourth heart surgery James made many

45

extra trips by the office to encourage us. James and Janet had been at our sides through each of Tom's other heart crises. The four of us had seen each others' children through teen-age angst and into successful young adulthood. We had shared good days and bad in the business and in our personal lives. Tom and I somewhat selfishly felt an emptiness knowing that they would be elsewhere while Tom lay on the operating table. James, tall and big, and with the voice to match, was in the habit of clasping an arm, a shoulder or even a knee when explaining a business point and saying, "Are you with me?" Grabbing both of us by our shoulders in a tight hug, James said he would see us after his vacation and after Tom's surgery. Squeezing our shoulders, James repeated with great conviction that he expected Tom's surgery to go well. It was as if our friend was willing a good outcome for Tom. Cigarette in hand James began the climb from the guest-house-office, past the pool, and up the slope to his truck. Midway he stopped to catch his breath. Tom hollered out to him, that he needed to see a cardiologist. James replied that he was fine; he had just had a physical. The two friends had exchanged similar words often in the months following Tom's third surgery. With a final wave, James finished the climb to his truck, put out his cigarette, and drove away. We did not see him again. Within a few days of Tom's release from the hospital after the fourth *cabbage*, we received word that James had gone to sleep after a day of sight-seeing and did not awaken on this earth again. Getting word of James's death hit Tom much harder than his own surgery had. It was hard for us both; we were devastated at the loss of our friend, and we hurt for his wife and family. Tom struggled for a long time with why he, with the broken heart, had been spared, and his dearest friend had been taken. The whys remain even now, less painful because we know that out of pain God works His plan. He knows the answers. He loves us, and He is in control. We know that we will rejoin our friend (and a host of other friends and family members) in due time. We would not be at all surprised when we arrive in God's presence to have James greet us there, grabbing our shoulders with those big hands. Instead of that trademark phrase, "Are you with me?" he will state, "Now you're with me...it just took you longer to get here."

Tom's fourth surgery was the third surgery done on him by Dr. Michael. Late in the afternoon after the arteriogram, after both the cardiologist and the surgeon had spoken with us, I wondered if there would be any material left in Tom's body to patch his ailing heart. The outlook was not promising. Although Dr. Michael had said that he would be able to use the right mammary artery to build the grafts Tom needed, we were aware that Tom's chances of recovery were certainly not as good as they had been with his earlier surgeries. We were both worried, both sad, both trying to put on a good front for the other. The hospital crew moved Tom to a windowless room in the coronary care unit. The coronary care nurses knew Tom pretty well after all the surgeries and procedures he had undergone. They knew he hated not having windows, so just in time for a spectacular springtime sunset two of them came to roll his bed to a room with a western facing window. The blue sky touched with red and gold, and the huge flaming orb going down was a vivid reminder of God's majesty. The beauty before me, the kindness shown us and the uncertainty facing us made it difficult for me to hold my tears until I could leave Tom's bedside. I squeezed my husband's hand, smiled unsteadily, and left the room as quickly as I could.

Once more Tom's surgery went well thanks to God's mercy and the surgeon's skill. When Tom was back in a room the nurses bent the rules so our three grandchildren, all toddlers, were able to see that their beloved Poppa Tom was going to recover. As young as the toddlers were, they were not immune to the anxiety oozing from the adults in the family. They decorated Tom's room with scribbled drawings; they sat on the edge of his bed to solemnly point at his scars and ask if his heart was still "thumping around in there." After another successful cabbage he could answer that indeed it was! Ben's, Hannah's and Samantha's visits were likely more healing for Tom than many of his medicines.

As in previous times the presence and prayers of family and friends had lifted us up, enabling us to get through dark days. Over a decade later our memories of their love and kindness stir our emotions as if the events had taken place recently. A friend recounts that during this time she recorded in her own journal that prayers were being spoken to lift us up in our battle just as Moses' arms had been lifted when his energy flagged. We felt that strength and energy and without it we would have struggled mightily. The loving actions of friends and family made us, unworthy as we are, know we are valued in their sight and in the sight of God.

We had become accustomed after four surgeries to uneventful recoveries, but that was about to change. Tom was discharged from the hospital with a small mass in his left groin. It was at the site where he had been attached to the heart-lung bypass machine during the surgery. The doctors expected it to become even smaller in the weeks to come. They sent my husband home with instructions to keep the site covered with a gauze bandage and to keep it clean.

When Dr. Michael came by to discharge Tom from the hospital, he told us that he was leaving for a mountain climbing vacation in South America. He had, in fact, been talking excitedly about this upcoming adventure even before Tom's surgery. We had a business friend who had been among the first climbers to conquer K2 in the Himalayas. Pete had given our son an autographed copy of a book written about his adventures, which Tad passed on to Dr. Michael as a token of our appreciation for the care he had given Tom. Dr. Michael was thrilled with the book. Thumbing through it as he walked out the door of the room, he said that if Tom had any problems he was to call his partner, Dr. Charles.

The first two weeks Tom was at home passed without a problem, but toward the end of that time the small mass in Tom's groin began to drain. The drainage became thick and yellow in a matter of days. My husband developed a fever. May 9, a Saturday, Tom was back at the hospital emergency room. We called our surgeon's partner, Dr. Charles, who knew my husband's history from having assisted in harvesting graft material from Tom's legs in several surgeries. When Dr. Charles came to the emergency room he said that the mass in Tom's groin was a contaminated lymphocele which would have to be removed. Tom had experienced small knots at the site of cannula entries before but none of them had become a problem. Most likely a lymph node had been nicked during surgery. This had allowed fluid to seep into the surrounding area and rather than re-absorbing it, the area had become infected. Tom spent Mother's Day in surgery having the mass removed and I spent the day back in the intensive care waiting room.

Between the two of us Tom and I have spent several holidays in the hospital. Early in our marriage I spent Valentine's Day, my October birthday and Thanksgiving hospitalized. Tom added our daughter's May birthday, Mother's Day, Father's Day, St. Patrick's Day, at least one wedding anniversary and Easter to our calendar. We can attest that holiday food does not taste as good in the hospital as it does at home. Speaking of food, there is also the saga of Tom's chicken dinner; during each hospitalization for his heart Tom was served, at least once, a very bland, skinless, unseasoned chicken breast for dinner. Since Tom never ate the chicken breast, it became a family joke that the dietician tagged it with his name, froze it, thawed it, and sent it back on his tray each time he was a patient.

48

Three days after the surgery to remove the lymphocele, with the wound packed and sterile, Dr Charles released Tom to go home saying that a visiting nurse would be by twice daily to change the dressing. Tom could not swim in our pool the entire summer, and his physical activity was quite limited until the groin wound healed. The site showed no signs of infection and appeared to be slowly healing. I am not squeamish, so the nurse taught me to change the dressings and came by less often to check my sterile technique and the progress Tom was making in healing. When I first began dressing the wound on my own, I could almost hide my hand in the hole that was there; needless to say it had to heal from the inside out. The lasting effect of the infected lymph node was that it left Tom with only one area, the right groin, for any future catheterizations. The scar it left did later cause one nurse helping him disrobe to utter, "Mein Gott, what did they do to you?" It is *not* a pretty scar.

After Tom's groin healed he had more treadmill tests to check the function level of his heart. The heart showed its battle scars; the ejection fraction, the organ's ability to pump, had fallen. The first treadmill was halted due to the patient's shortness of breath. In a couple of months when Tom was stronger he did a thallium treadmill study. The radioisotopes, giving a more precise reading, showed similar results.

January 1999, approximately eight and a half months after his fourth bypass surgery, Tom's regularly scheduled stress echocardiogram was done. The report talks about the heart becoming *dyskinetic*-not moving properly, and dysfunctional due to ischemic heart disease. There was that word again, the one that Tom refused to internalize. He had a *disease* and it continued to damage his heart. Whether or not Tom was willing to hear that word, the facts were that his heart muscle did not move properly, and it did not function as a healthy heart would. By February Tom had increasing angina, and another heart cath was scheduled. The results were not encouraging. The left anterior descending artery was one hundred percent blocked. On the right, two of the grafts were each one hundred percent blocked; the other grafts were sixty and forty percent occluded. This test also told us that Tom's mitral valve was no longer functioning properly, meaning that blood was regurgitated into the wrong cavity of the heart.

Recollecting these years Tom and I are struck by our attitudes between our bouts with this progressive disease. Certainly we were aware of the problems with Tom's heart and that they had only worsened in spite of all efforts. At some level our lives did revolve around our fear of the *what-ifs*, but for blocks of time there were other things that claimed first priority in our minds. We continued to wrestle with business issues, but we also enjoyed life. We watched in wonder as our grandchildren grew from toddlers into children with distinctly different personalities and interests. We enjoyed good times with dear friends. We lost parents and grieved. Our lives were as mundane and as magical as most lives are, and all around us we were becoming increasingly more aware of the over-stretching love of God, the Father, even in the worst of times. Becoming aware of God's love does not mean that we always heard or heeded His voice when He called. I like to think that God (with a little help from one of Leigh's friends) had some fun with Tom about not listening. It was a warm day and Tom was working on a project. All the pieces of the machinery, which was not functioning as he wanted it to, were spread on the triple carport. The task was not going well and Tom got vocal. The air may not have turned blue as he muttered his displeasure, but I suspect there was a tint of azure. No sooner had an oath passed Tom's lips than he heard an ethereal voice quite clearly call his name. Dropping the wrench he held in his hand, Tom turned toward the driveway, expecting to see someone standing there. No one was there, but again he clearly heard his name wafting through the air. Peering first toward our neighbors' yard and then toward the pool and guesthouse, Tom could not see a soul. With a sheepish grin on his face, my husband came into the kitchen to joke that maybe God was calling his name, and that just maybe he should watch his language more carefully. As it turned out, our daughter's friend, Allison, had been floating over our house in a hot air balloon and had enjoyed playing this prank on Tom. Maybe God just used Allison's fun-loving nature to vividly illustrate that He had been repeatedly calling Tom's name-and that it was time to listen up.

9

To Arms, Two Arms

Early in 1999, Tom, exhausted because of his malfunctioning heart, was again experiencing chest pain. The results of the latest arteriogram were dismal. Tom needed surgery. He had no more mammary arteries. His saphenous veins front and back, had been used. Stents did not last in his heart. Medicines were no longer getting the job done. Dr. Drew wanted a couple of days to consider our shrinking options. Saying that he and Dr. Michael would confer, he sent us home with a promise to be in touch early in the following week. He admonished Tom to severely limit his activities because of his badly damaged heart.

Our city is a small one. You run into folks out shopping, in restaurants and around town. Our paths and those of our physicians crossed frequently. Sunday morning Dr. Michael, Tom and I all attended the same service at our church. I remember as we were leaving the sanctuary that blustery morning that Dr. Michael grabbed Tom's shoulder and said something like, "Man, we've got one chance to fix this, but it hasn't been done here yet." Dr. Michael has the sort of contagious enthusiasm that buoys your spirits and makes you believe that the impossible might just be possible after all. Talking a moment in front of the church he told us that there were a couple of more articles he wanted to read and a cardiovascular surgeon or two, one of them a cousin of Tom's, whose brains he wanted to pick. Dr. Michael wanted our family all together when he set out the possibilities before us. Our daughter and her family were living in the same town as we. Our son was serving in an Air Force hospital in Texas. He and his family

51

had been home for Christmas but were more than willing to make the ten hour drive again with their two young children.

The following Sunday morning Dr. Michael, as good as his word, pulled into the circle driveway in front of our house. I had a pot of coffee ready, so with full cups in hand we gathered in our living room to hear what the doctor had to say. He told us that a surgery using the arteries in the arms for coronary bypass material was being done. As I recall, Dr. Michael said that some Australian physicians had done it and had presented a paper on their results. He had copies of the article to share with us all, but particularly with our physician son. Dr. Michael told us that although this particular surgery had not been done in our town, and although he had not done one, he felt that after reading the material, studying it and discussing it with colleagues that it was a surgery he could do. I remember that he and our son made the old medical joke about *see one, do one, teach one* with my husband joining in the laughter before the conversation turned serious.

Dr. Michael said that he was aware that the fact that he had no experience with this particular surgery might mean that Tom and the family would be more comfortable going elsewhere. He said he would be fine if we chose that option. We discussed several of the large heart centers in the United States, including the Cleveland Clinic in Ohio, where this technique had been done. We family members knew that a decision needed to be reached quickly. The likelihood of Tom's suffering a fatal myocardial infarction increased daily. We had hard questions to ask, and we knew we would hear equally hard answers. Dr. Michael stated what we all already knew, that Tom's chances of surviving this surgery were less than they had been for the other four chest crackings. We, the family, danced around the edges of the ramifications of that statement without saying much. I remembered the evening the CVICU nurses had moved Tom to a room with a window so that he could see one last magnificent sunset, and how slim I had considered his chances then. Yet here we were, only months later, in a more serious situation. My mind recoiled from hearing actual percentages put to Tom's chance for survival. Our son's face was solemn as he struggled to maintain control of his emotions. Looking at Tad's face only confirmed my assumption that Tom's chances would be poor, and my soul shriveled within me. Just then I heard Leigh ask Dr. Michael why he thought her dad's chances would not be as good, and exactly what sort of survival rate was he talking about. No more dancing around the issue and the foray into the center of it had come, unexpectedly, from the baby of the family. A little taken aback, Dr. Michael turned to face Leigh, and with that charming grin, said to her, "Whew, you ask the hard stuff!" The icy grip fear had on us relaxed in a pool of self-conscious chuckles. Dr, Michael then gave Leigh and the rest of us the hard answers we had to hear. Tom's chances for survival were no better than ten percent. Even so, those odds were better than the ones he faced without intervention. The coffee in our cups was cold; conversation lagged. Dr. Michael had been generous with his time-it is not every day that a heart surgeon makes a house call. He had answered every question we had been able to think of asking. His answers had been unequivocal and honest. Our gazes all fell on Tom. Ultimately the decision, even though the family had been included in the discussion, was his. It was Tom's body, his disease, and his percent of a chance to either live or die. Looking his surgeon straight in the eye Tom said that since Dr. Michael had been the one to open his chest three previous times; he wanted him, since he was willing , to be the surgeon for this fifth operation. In Tom's words Dr. Michael knew where the *shrapnel*, the scars, and the trouble spots were in a way that a new surgeon could not comprehend. It was settled. Dr. Michael would attempt to repair my husband's heart for the fifth time using arteries he would harvest from Tom's arms. Giving hugs all round, and still teasing Leigh about asking the hard questions, Dr. Michael went toward our heavy, wooden front doors. He said that Tom would need an arteriogram of the arteries in his arms to see if they were suitable for the surgery. He would schedule that, and be in touch with us. The front doors closed behind Dr. Michael. We watched his truck pull out the driveway then silence swallowed the room as we each retreated into our own private thoughts about what lay ahead.

Dr. Michael scheduled the arteriogram of Tom's radial arteries for March 3. This test proved that in Tom's arms the ulnar artery was dominant and would leave him with sufficient circulation in his arms and hands. Each of us has in our arms more than one set of arteries, another fail-safe backup provided by God's incredible design. These are the brachial, radial, ulnar and interosseous. Coursing through the vessels in my husband's arms, the dye revealed complete arches of the radial arteries at the hands indicating that using those arteries for bypass grafts could be tolerated. Prior to Tom's trip to the hospital, as different friends and church groups prayed for him and for our family, the fact that Dr. Michael would be doing a surgery not yet done in our town got innocently embellished. By the time we heard about the surgery again, it had become an *experimental procedure,* rather like the childhood game of *Gossip* where a phrase is whispered in the ear of the person next to you, and so on around until it returns to the point of origin sounding nothing like what it started as. Our surprise was nothing compared to Dr. Michael's when he heard that he would be doing *experimental* surgery on Tom.

I cannot write this without picturing Tom's body with all its scars. Imagine the midline scar on his chest, opened four times, soon to be five; the bilateral scars at his groin, one a deep, pulled hollow, the scars running the length of his legs, front and back. This was the body of the man I loved, had walked beside, raised children with; it was infinitely precious to me. How could I stand to see it scarred still more? How could I bear for them to lay open his arms, the arms that had held me, and had held our babies? How could his body withstand one more insult? Yet, how could I not encourage this surgery that seemed our only option for a continued life together?

Within a week Tom was admitted to the hospital for his fifth coronary artery bypass surgery. All of us were dismally aware of its high risk. On the eve of the surgery our children arranged for us to go as their guests to our favorite restaurant where chef and staff treated us to a gourmet meal, fine wine, and excellent service. Tom would be entering the hospital the following morning through the outpatient department again. This method of being admitted to the hospital seemed strange since our situation was so critical. Still we were grateful for this last evening of pretend normalcy, trying to keep the mood light, even celebratory. We wanted good memories. Knowing that sleep would evade us both, we had rented several movies planning to stay cuddled on the couch the entire night watching them. In the early morning hours we gave that up, switched off the television, and crawled into bed too tense to sleep and too tired to stay up longer. We lay in silence, each wrapped in his private thoughts. Tom has not shared his thoughts during those pre-dawn, pre-surgery hours. When pressed, he admits to fear although he thinks he displaced those thoughts by wondering about the process, the procedure the surgeon would use as he harvested the arteries. I cannot imagine having the courage to face the surgeon's knife for the fifth time. I remember praying silently for Tom, for the family to be strong in whatever we faced. I do not think I prayed for God's will to be done. I had not developed a faith of that depth. Our faith journey, Tom's and mine, was not, as I have already said, a steady climb over the boulders in our path. We wavered and waffled, though not always at the same time, as we found our footing. At times we slogged through swamps of despair and deserts of doubt. God was present in all of that whether we always recognized Him or not. There is an old prayer that is attributed to St. Patrick which says something like this-*Christ before me, Christ beside me, Christ behind me.* Thus, according to legend, St. Patrick prayed for protection as he walked into the wilds of Ireland and the unknown. Tom and I did not voice that prayer, but surely our souls must have wordlessly moaned it, and hearing the cries of our hearts, the sweet Holy Spirit did surround us-always.

Before dawn March 9, we checked into the hospital through the ambulatory surgery center, grateful that we had been allowed to spend a last night together in our own home. Many of the staff and nurses remembered us from Tom's previous surgeries and procedures. A few who now worked in other parts of the hospital came by to wish Tom well or to give us hugs. They made things as easy for us as they were able. When the attendants came for Tom I walked with his gurney as far as the surgery holding area, kissed him good-bye, and heard him tell me he'd see me in a few hours. I stumbled toward the waiting room, the tears I could shed once out of his sight blurring my vision. In the years we had been making these trips the waiting room had been moved from that cold, windy spot on the first floor to a large space in an upper story. Also, I no longer got lost traveling the halls of coronary care. I had, unfortunately, lots of experience finding my way through that labyrinth.

Spacious as it was, the waiting room was very full even in those pre-dawn hours. The crowd divided itself into two camps with each group occupying an end of the long room. I haven't words to describe the slowness with which time passed that day. Tom went to surgery before sunrise; I did not see him again until well after sunset. With enervating tedium the day wore on. Periodically, Dr. Michael would call the hostess's desk; I would be called to the phone and he would tell me things were going well. I lived for those calls. By afternoon the two groups in the waiting room had, as people often do, made a connection. Although we had not known each other, the family of the other patient lived not far from our neighborhood; that patient, like Tom, had been a Scoutmaster and they had at least a nodding acquaintance through those activities. That family included grown children waiting with their mother as their father fought for his life against a disease as frightening as Tom's heart disease. Over the next several days when the numbers of our two groups waned, we visited with and consoled each other.

I do not know the exact number of hours and minutes this non-experimental, but most extraordinary surgery took but more than eight hours passed before Dr. Michael came to the waiting area to talk to us. Part of what he said I did not immediately grasp. I heard only that Tom had tolerated the surgery well and was in recovery. Dr. Michael, looking more tired than I had ever seen him look, but smiling broadly, hugged each of us. He commented jokingly that had this operation not gone well, he might have hung it up. Dr. Michael explained that Tom had required three grafts; a fourth had been considered and rejected due to a lack of suitable material to construct it. A Carpentier ring had been placed in Tom's mitral valve to help it to open and close properly. Dr. Michael further explained that the brachial arteries have many small vessels running from them, and that each of those tiny bleeders had to be painstakingly tied off before moving on to the next. Once the arteries were removed they had a tendency to spasm. In order to lessen that problem, Dr. Michael and his team had soaked the arteries in a solution to relax them before constructing the grafts. The doctor did admit to a slight concern that one of his lungs might have stuck to the chest wall due to the nature of the surgery, and the texture of Tom's organs from the wear and tear of his disease, and all of his previous surgeries. Dr. Michael wanted to monitor that closely; otherwise he reported that he was well pleased with the way this fifth surgery had gone. Relief washed over me with the force of a tsunami. I wept.

Remarkably, it was not until after this fifth surgery that Tom needed a blood transfusion and platelets. I was not a suitable donor but friends, church members, people that we barely knew from the community, joined our children in donating this gift of life. The experience gave a face to every Red Cross blood drive I would hear advertised from that day to this. Seven days after this high risk surgery Tom went home. The discharge summary calls his recovery uneventful and his post-op course essentially unremarkable. Those adjectives may suit what had transpired medically, but to our family this surgery was, save the births of our children and grandchildren, the most remarkable thing that we had ever experienced. Tom was at home a week and a day when, suffering from a high fever and shortness of breath, he was re-admitted to the hospital for anemia and pleural effusion, fluid around his lung. He was given a unit and a half of blood to which he had an allergic reaction. Dr. Michael started steroids immediately. Tom had been released from the hospital after his fifth surgery taking a prescribed blood thinner, Coumadin, to ease the load on his recovering heart. With fluid pressing on his heart and lungs and causing him difficulty breathing, the doctors needed to tap his chest. They could not insert a tube into his chest cavity until the effects of the anticoagulant had been reversed. The Coumadin was stopped, and Tom was given doses of vitamin K. When the physicians were at last able to tap Tom's chest, two liters of fluid were drawn from it. He improved dramatically and was released to go home once more. A second tap had to be done before Tom turned the corner toward regaining his health. Within a month or so x-rays showed a much smaller effusion still present, mainly on the left side of Tom's chest, but at this point Tom's recovery *did* become uneventful. Once more we were indebted to God's grace and the physicians' skill for Tom's life.

As we approach events in the not so far distant past, the story becomes more difficult, more painful to recall and to put on paper. I, more than Tom, find reasons to avoid facing it all again. He insists that is because he always slept through the really hard parts. I think my reluctance to share all our story stems from something more complex-a combination of weakness and misplaced pride. I am not wise in the ways of spiritual warfare, but I sometimes think this is Satan's effort to stymie the glory we would give God for the mercy and grace He continues to bestow upon us.

While Tom was recuperating, our office remained in our guest house. On one of those days a second friend knocked on our door offering to help with the business. A retired accountant with a law degree, he was way over-qualified for the job. I do not know why God gave Tom and me such extraordinary, loving friends to help us in our struggles, but He did and we praise Him for them. William stepped in at a time when my parents were requiring more care. His help was invaluable. Tom's recovery eventually would enable us to move the office back to the same property with the manufacturing plant. While he continued recuperating though, our bookkeeping operations remained in the guesthouse. As William and I worked there one day he unwittingly made a statement that indicated to me Tom continued to be less than forthcoming about the economic situation in which we were becoming mired. My reaction was to do what I always did and that was to run-this time literally. I was devastated that after all we had faced, my husband still would not share bad business news with me. Fighting back tears, I got my dog, got in my car and sped out of town. William had spoken in innocence. I reacted childishly. I don't know who other only children, including us grown up ones, talk to when they are hurt; I have always talked to my dog. They look at you with understanding eyes; they love you unconditionally; they expect little other than a pat on the head and a bit of dinner, and they lick away your salty tears. So my dog, Angel, an Old English Sheep Dog, and I put the pedal to the metal and fled to a small lake west of town. We walked through the campsites out onto a concrete platform in the middle of the lake. Meanwhile back in town our friend, William, fearing I was upset enough to harm myself, called our minister. I must have appeared even more frazzled than I really was, and due to recent tragic events in our circle of friends, suicides were on all our minds. Tom returned from the plant to the chaos his behavior had generated. Pretty certain that he knew about where I would be, my husband set out to find me. As the afternoon shadows lengthened, I sat on that platform over the lake with my Angel beside me trying to process my anger and my feelings of betrayal. I considered running further but had little money and no credit cards with me. I didn't think rationally. I behaved childishly. I did not claim my part in the situation Tom and I had built. My problem was that I kept talking to my sheep dog and not the Shepherd.

We heard the car drive up, Angel and I, and she ran to greet Tom. I sure wasn't that glad to see him. He apologized with what I had come to view as the standard *I was protecting you* speech. He made what I knew were empty promises that this sort of deception would never happen again. I should have stiffened my spine and seen our confrontation through to a healthy conclusion, but still seething with thinly veiled anger, and full of distrust, I agreed to return to the city. Tom got into his car feeling that he'd won the argument. Maybe inside himself he admitted that he had violated a trust, but I don't think so. Haggard, tear-stained, and emotionally wrung out, I got home to learn that I needed to let our minister know I was okay. Embarrassed, I called. It took a while to look the minister in the eye again, and to realize that I was blessed to have a friend like William, caring enough to try to help me when he thought I was beyond helping myself.

Tom moved the office back to our factory. I was more out of the daily machinations of the business than I had been at any point since we had started it. My observation was that Tom was increasingly less excited about his work. He didn't have the energy reserves he'd once had. The business climate was more difficult. We had made some major errors in judgment and were losing ground economically. After my run away Tom did share, guardedly, some of the worsening financial information with me. Together we put the majority of our personal savings into the business because we felt we owed it to our employees and because Tom could not say we needed to get out, and I would not say it. As was my history, I accepted the information Tom shared without question. As was his history, he continued to share financial information with me in a selective manner.

The loss of two friends during this period hit Tom hard. His business friend with similar symptoms died. He had finished a large architectural project in our city. We had talked with him at its grand opening when he admitted to Tom that he was not feeling well. A short time later he was hospitalized, the arteries from his arms were harvested for grafts but his condition after surgery worsened. The decision to send him to the Cleveland Clinic for transplant was made. He was flown there, but due to multiple complications he did not live long enough to receive a heart. Tom and I were at his funeral in a church he had designed. There were people standing in every available space, even in the areas adjacent to the sanctuary. In New England an old friend, one we both admired for her warm heart and her wit, died of a brain aneurysm. I was needed at home, but Tom flew up for the funeral and to be with her husband. Out of the pain of their loss, Suellen's husband and adult children did as she wanted and gave the gift of a better life to multiple organ recipients. Once again, just as it had with my cousin's transplant years earlier, the idea of organ donation and receipt crept to the edge of our consciousness.

10

After Taking the Fifth

The expected Y2K crisis passed with a fizzle. Even Tom's heart seemed to be functioning in a reasonably steady manner. Tad, Leigh and I understood, though we rarely discussed it, that Tom's heart was failing. Tom never voiced that recognition. The elephant still lived in our rooms. By the third quarter of the year 2000 Tom was back in the hospital as an outpatient for an electrical conduction study of his heart and a stress echocardiogram. Prior to this time Tom's problems with his heart had been with the plumbing; now his electrical system was compromised. According to the records, his problem was moderately severe and worsened with exercise. He got a pacemaker. His angina was categorized as Class II, and even in the physician's notes there is recognition that emotional stress was at least as damaging for Tom as physical stress. Cold weather, especially windy weather, was hard on Tom. He was at last on a regular schedule of exercise.

2001 brought no major health crises for Tom, just a slow decline in stamina and an increase in angina. Our physician convinced Tom that it was time to apply for disability. That was, in many ways, a demoralizing step for my husband. He continued to put in an appearance at the plant when he was able. It was long past time to get out of the business, but still Tom held on. He hadn't the strength to give our business the time and energy it needed. He had not trained or hired personnel to take up the slack. I stepped away from the business more as the months rolled by because my mother was dealing with Alzheimer's, and she and my dad needed my help. Had the business been the patient it would have been relegated to intensive care. Instead of being wise and closing the plant, we agreed to pour more of our own funds from savings and insurance policies into it. I agreed to the plan although it was, in retrospect, the worst possible decision we could have made. We did it partly, I suppose, as a matter of pride. We didn't want to be quitters; we didn't want to let down the people who worked for us. Our actions did not give our business the breath of life; they prolonged the throes of its death.

In the spring of 2002 our long-time cardiologist and friend had taken a sabbatical. Tom noticed what he described as palpitations or a racing heart beat. When he could no longer ignore this change in his heart, Tom called for an appointment with a new partner in that practice. Their personalities did not mesh. Admittedly, it would have been difficult for anyone to measure up in Tom's estimation to the doctor who had been treating him for twenty years. 2002 was a tough year. My mother died in June. Shortly thereafter my beloved sheepdog and confidant, Angel, died. It was obvious that Tom was losing ground and that he needed the attention of a cardiologist. He was fatigued and having chest pain with exertion. There was a bright, young doctor, not long in private practice, who was a friend of our son's and who had been in Tom's Scout troop. Feeling a bit guilty for burdening the doctor with caring for someone he had known long and well, Tom called for an appointment. Dr. Anthony graciously assumed his care knowing that when Dr. Drew came back to his practice Tom would return to him.

Dr. Anthony talked with us about the limited options that we had for treating Tom. It was decided after reviewing information gleaned from Tom's wearing a Holter monitor that the best plan would be to pursue more aggressive drug therapy. Dr. Anthony spoke very plainly to us both about the possibility of sudden cardiac death in view of the significant area of scarring on the walls of Tom's heart. In addition to changes in medications, the cardiologist wanted Tom to attend cardiac rehabilitation, and to try an eight week course of EECP.

EECP stands for *enhanced external counter pulsation*, an induced counter beat or pulse which attempts to optimize small vessel or collateral flow to the coronary arteries. For this treatment, one that had been practiced in China for a couple of decades, the patient wore a suit similar to a jet pilot's G-suit. Sensors in the suit reacted to the heartbeat of the patient causing an artificial pulsation while the actual heart was at rest. This double pressure was meant to dilate the smaller vessels, thus increasing the blood flow to the heart. Tom went every day for this treatment. For the first several times I accompanied him. On Tom's first visit Dr. Newman, the physician running the clinic, examined Tom and explained the process to him. Nurses helped get my husband into a suit which sort of resembled coveralls. They positioned him on a table in a room full of three or four such tables occupied by other patients. They then allowed me to sit in a straight-backed chair beside him. From the beginning, Tom appeared to be getting a violent pounding by this machine. The nurses said that he would become accustomed to it. They explained the principle of counterpulsation to us again. Suggesting that Tom read a magazine or book to take his mind from the throbbing machine, they left the room. Because Tom's body was being jerked around so much the idea of reading something was ludicrous. It was impossible to talk above the noise the machines made. Periodically someone would check on Tom as he thrashed about the table and would assure us that he was doing fine. I stopped the machine several times that first visit; I thought it was malfunctioning. Eventually, I simply brought Tom to these sessions and picked him up. I could not stand watching the beating he was taking. Since the EECP sensors functioned by running off the patient's heartbeat, the machine was fooled by Tom's PVC's, extra beats, into firing too often. This was what was causing it to pummel Tom. Four weeks into the treatment, still thinking that surely things would improve, and knowing that his options were limited; Tom kept a second appointment with Dr. Anthony. They decided it was time to further assist the electrical system of Tom's heart. Although he had worn a pacemaker for quite awhile, tests indicated that he needed a defibrillator. My husband's severely compromised heart was always one beat away from instant cardiac death.

An electrophysiologist, removing the old device, inserted a combined pacemaker/defibrillator just below Tom's collarbone on the left side. Even with this device, Tom fared no better in the EECP clinic. His heart continued to spark extra beats which in turn caused the machine to pound him relentlessly. Tom endured thirty-five of these tortuous sessions with a stiff-upper-lip tenacity. The final visit he was in severe pain when he got up from the table, and he was too weak to walk to the car. He sat in the waiting room until he could leave under his own power. Frustrated with their previous responses, Tom did not share his suspicions that he had suffered a heart attack with the nurses. Since this was one of the few days I had not taken him to his appointment, he eventually drove himself home. He did not share his suspicions with Dr. Anthony or with me. If

Tom suffered another heart attack that day, thank God it did not lead to sudden death.

In June Tom was back in the hospital in order for the electrophysiologist to shock him. Medicine had failed to control his atrial flutter, leading to *tachycardia*-a runaway heart beat. The physician used electrical shock to cardiovert the heart back to a more desirable rhythm. Tom returned to his room with a burn on his back that looked as if someone had held a hot iron there. The heart's beat had been changed with a single jolt of 120 joules. Although Tom was still in heart failure he did not have the fatigue or the difficulty breathing that he had experienced when his heart was not in sinus rhythm. By early October, Tom had completed the EECP therapy, but was still attending rehabilitation sessions at the local hospital. Physically he had lost no more ground. Anxiety over the business, however, was preventing his sleeping well at night. He was constantly fatigued. Toward the end of that month Dr. Anthony sent Tom to the hospital for more tests. After registering through the outpatient department we were waiting to be called when we noticed a familiar face in a group of people seated nearby. It was our old friend and cardiologist, Dr. Drew. It was an odd moment, our seeing him as a visitor to the hospital rather than as a physician, and his seeing Tom there for an appointment instigated by someone other than himself. As Dr. Drew questioned Tom about his condition, you could almost see the wheels turning in his head reviewing the twenty years of my husband's heart history. Dr. Drew's parting comment was that he would see Tom in his office the following day. With gratitude, and with his blessing, we left Dr. Anthony and went home to Dr. Drew.

The following, fateful October day we waited in Dr. Drew's familiar office. We heard the death sentence; there was nothing more the doctor could do. Finally everyone, even Tom, had to acknowledge the elephant in the room. Oddly enough it was almost exactly twenty years from the date of Tom's first heart attack. Dr. Drew presented the possibility of a transplant. Tom initially refused and then agreed to consider the transplant option. Stunned and silent we left the office to go home, to talk with our family, to pray, and to try to sort out our meager possibilities.

11

Heart Failure Clinic

Tom began treatment at the heart failure clinic in the same hospital where he had experienced every heart surgery and every procedure. Perhaps it was appropriate that his first appointment was October 31, 2002-*Halloween*. It felt as if there were demons and a few ghosts stalking us. Many of the details of this time in our journey are blurred for us both. For Tom it was a struggle simply to breathe. Most nights he was in a recliner rather than a bed and during daylight hours he was often in the same chair without the energy to be elsewhere. He was losing weight at a dramatic rate; he lacked the desire or the energy to eat. His complexion was either pale or gray. His thoughts were sometimes foggy because the blood supply to his brain was poor and oxygen-starved. If I had been, as our daughter described, on auto-pilot, early in our struggle with heart disease, I am not sure how to describe my emotional state at this point; the word that comes to mind is *numb*; I was numb. Perhaps some psychiatrist might say I was suffering from something akin to post-traumatic stress syndrome. I don't know because I never saw a doctor. I made one attempt to talk to a counselor, but decided that was money wasted when I found myself telling her what she wanted to hear to be able to say that I was handling the stress in a healthy manner. I felt like a punching bag. Each time I bounced back there was a heart surgery; there was my mother's death; there were other crises just as monumental that have no place in this story. Underneath it all was my unspoken anxiety about our economic situation. The business was in dire need of firm management. Neither of us was able to give it

65

that and no one else was in place to take over. Perhaps the people working there did the best they could; I would like to think so. True to our history Tom and I talked little about our situation. I wanted to protect him from facts and criticisms that he was too ill to face. Down deep I did not want to hear the facts either since in some way I felt that hearing them would be disloyal to Tom. I hauled out the lipstick and the smile that over the years had as many resurrections as Tom's plate full of skinless, colorless, tasteless chicken reportedly served up by the dietician during each of his hospital stays.

On his first day as a heart failure patient Tom met an angel disguised as an RN. Her name was Nori. If not for her ministrations and those of her colleague, Margie, it would have been practically impossible for Tom to view the heart failure clinic as little more than a waiting room for death. Think about it-here is a man who with each episode and ensuing repair has told himself that he was cured; here is a fighter who had often gotten by on pure grit and determination; here is a man who had always believed that he was in charge of his own destiny. Now he was forced to face his mortality. He was in control of very little of his future. Death was at times a more real possibility than life. In those days the heart failure clinic was located on the hospital's ground floor near the area where we had so often checked in for Tom's surgeries. It was a long room with several recliners, a round table and chairs, and the usual cabinets for supplies. There were a couple of televisions. There was little privacy in those pre-HIPPA (Health Information Patient Privacy Act) days. We met the nurses; I stayed with Tom that first day. After taking his history, Nori started two IV's, one was a newer drug and the other was dopamine. The medicines were to ease the load on Tom's heart, to keep him alive. Through the first three weeks of November Tom went to the Heart Failure Clinic once a week; each visit lasted five hours and each time he received two IV's of the same drugs he had been given during his first appointment. Nori and Margie spent time during each visit reinforcing ways Tom could maintain as he waited for transplant evaluation. With the medicine he was receiving Tom was able to sleep better, actually spending some nights in the bed.

Due in part to the events of September 11, 2001 our daughter and granddaughter were back in Arkansas and living with us. They had come home for what was to have been a visit but our daughter had been hospitalized with viral meningitis. Her recovery was long and difficult and when she was unable to return to her job as a pre-school teacher that fall, they stayed on. Eventually she found work here and also started classes. I

66

was trying to work some at our factory as well as help my aging father, who was still grieving the loss of my mother, his wife of sixty two years. Dad's health was not great. He continued to live in our guesthouse but to take at least one meal a day with us. There were times during teacher work days and holidays when our granddaughter had no choice but to accompany Tom to the heart failure clinic. She and Nori became friends and on one particular visit she received a gift of fancy little socks with handmade edging from Nori. She was so excited that she tried to wear them every day. Nori's care embraced us all, not just her patient. After every visit to the clinic Tom would remark on the kindness and concern shown by his nurses, not just to him, but to all the patients. Without privacy the patients were pretty much forced to watch the program choice of whoever claimed the television control first. Tom remembers, none too fondly, one patient who liked talk shows, certainly not his favorite, played at top volume. Firmly but kindly Margie and Nori adjusted the sound much to the delight of Tom and another gentleman with whom he had become friends. Tom's talking buddy was a dairyman just as my husband's father had been, so the two of them had a common thread for conversation. Not long into the treatment Tom's friend's visits stopped abruptly. Still not having come to terms with the logical end of heart failure, Tom questioned Nori about the dairyman's whereabouts. Nori busied herself with other patients and did her best to avoid an answer. At last she had to tell Tom that his friend had died. My husband was visibly shaken and depressed for some time after. The nurses worked so hard to keep their patients spirits up that I've no doubt it hurt them as much to reveal the truth as it hurt Tom to hear it. Tom opened up to those two gentle women, especially Nori, and began to voice some of his anxieties and concerns. The struggle just to dress himself, and to go through any semblance of an ordinary day was taking its toll. Tom was losing weight again. By the end of November he admitted to Nori that he was just tired.

Everyone came home for Thanksgiving. Our grandchildren now numbered four with the youngest just over a year old. I love to cook for the family as had my mother before me. When she had become too feeble for those chores I had assumed her mantle. This Thanksgiving, however, our children talked me into purchasing most of our dishes from a caterer. It just seemed wrong, but then everything seemed out of kilter during that time. The weather, at least, was beautiful, and the trees in our backyard still had golden leaves. We decided that we wanted a family portrait, one that would include four generations from my father through the grandchildren.

Weighing heavily on all our minds was the probability that without drastic change this would be our last holiday together; our last family portrait to include Tom, and possibly my father. The arrangements were made and Thanksgiving afternoon the photographer set up his equipment on our deck. Between attempts to get everyone smiling at the same time, we would rush Tom back into the house to prevent his becoming too chilled. He was being a good sport; he knew how much the children and I wanted the portrait and he probably knew why. It was clear that Tom was tired and that the rest of us were getting a little tense. The photographer hustled us onto the deck for the third or fourth try. Off to the side I heard our mild mannered and soft spoken daughter-in-law say through gritted teeth to the one child who would not smile, "We are a happy family. You will smile or I will spank you." It worked; we got a good picture at last.

November 27 was a cold day and a difficult one for Tom. The frigid air hurt him. The electrocardiogram done that visit showed that his heart was constantly paced. It was no longer maintaining proper rhythm even part of the time without a mechanical assist. He talked with the nurses about the possibility of being evaluated soon at the Cleveland Clinic for placement on the transplant list. His disease progressed relentlessly. The cardiologist decided that he should receive treatment every third day, still two medications, still two IV's and still for five hours at a time. At last we got our first calls and letters from Renee, the specialty nurse for the pre-transplant patients at the Cleveland Clinic. She joined Nori and Margie as one of Tom's team of encouragers. I did not meet her for several weeks, but each time I came home from work when she had called, Tom seemed to be encouraged. The same pall hung over our Christmas plans that had shaped our Thanksgiving holiday. What if this was our last Christmas together? That possibility had never seemed more real.

Nori, as she had gotten to know Tom better, had begun to treat his spiritual, along with his physical well being. She rarely let a session pass without talking to him about God's love for us and the mercy He shows us. The talks most often ended with the two of them holding hands and with Nori praying in her softly accented voice. She offered a life raft that Tom clung to. On Tom's second or third December visit Nori introduced him to a heart recipient she had been telling him about. Dorothy was a small, attractive African-American woman who had recently received a heart in St. Louis. Still recuperating, Dorothy tired easily but she visited with Tom for over an hour answering his questions, telling him about her experience and, like Nori, holding his hands and praying with him. Dorothy knew that her second chance at life was a God-given gift too precious to waste. She felt called to serve by sharing her story. When I picked Tom up from his session that day, he was more encouraged than I had seen him since he had enrolled in the heart failure clinic. He relayed what Dorothy had told him about her own transplant experience, and he said that she had agreed to return to the clinic in a few days to share her story with our family and to answer our questions.

Renee called from Cleveland to tell Tom that an evaluation packet was in the mail. His appointment for tests was to be December 18. Tom and I made plans to fly up alone. Leigh would stay at home caring for my father and her daughter and attending class. Our son would drive after work to Nashville from Memphis where he and his family lived, in order to get a late flight to Cleveland. He would meet us at our hotel on the campus of the Cleveland Clinic. I was so thankful Tad would be there to talk with and to hear what the doctors would say.

Dorothy came again to the Heart Failure Clinic to talk with our family. With her calm demeanor, her obvious faith and her prayers for us, she buoyed our spirits and gave us hope. Tom had continued to lose weight; it was now difficult to get a good IV stick in his arms and his *pulse ox* reading was low, another indicator that his worn out heart was barely functioning. On December 17, 2002, just hours before our flight to Cleveland, Tom made an extra trip to the heart failure clinic in the hope of getting enough medicine in his system to keep him going until we returned home.

12

The Evaluation

The drive to the airport and the flight to Cleveland were laden with equal measures of hope and fear. We had only carry-on luggage which I was handling. Tom protested that he could help with it when we both knew that he could not. We were anxious about what we would learn in Ohio. Christmas was in two weeks, and the threat of sudden cardiac death was very much on our minds. Somewhere in the mix of my concerns was anxiety over my Christmas shopping. Had I gotten something for each grandchild? I was stressed enough that without the presents laid out in front of me, I was not sure. On the flight Tom slept and I worried. The Cleveland airport is a little distance from the city, and the route our cab followed was neither scenic nor encouraging. Empty, deteriorating, factory buildings lined either side of the highway, silent sentinels saluting the fallen economy of the factory-laden mid-western rust belt. Dusk was approaching; the winter sky was gray; the buildings seen from the moving windows of our cab as we came to the city limits were gray and drab. The momentary triumph I had felt at successfully hailing a cab and getting Tom, our luggage and myself into it was fading. Since I was unfamiliar with Cleveland, I could only pray we were going in the right direction by the shortest route.

The Cleveland Clinic is an island of hope, technology and healing under almost constant construction in a neighborhood that ranges from severely depressed and depressing to homes that are being purchased and gentrified as people re-discover the charm of the architecture of the late

1800's and early 1900's. Tom and I were registered at a hotel on the hospital campus. The cab let us out right at the door of the Intercontinental. At that time two hotels were on the campus; I think there are now at least three. We had been registered at the less expensive of the two but because it was full, the hospital put us in the Intercontinental for the same price. One of the first things I noticed when we arrived was the international mix of the people staying at the Intercontinental. The hotel's guests were from everywhere and a trip through the lobby to the elevator brought several languages to one's ear. I had not expected this in Cleveland, Ohio but it was my first visit to a world class health center.

Tom was ashen, cold, and exhausted. We went to our room, a suite with a small kitchenette, where we rested and waited for our son to arrive. We knew that Tad had planned to leave Memphis after putting in a full day at the hospital, but we did not know that he had miscalculated the time his journey would require because he had forgotten that the Nashville airport was on the opposite side of town from Memphis. He barely made his flight. When he checked in and got to the room he noted with concern, his dad's pallor and general weakness. We ordered dinner in but Tom ate very little. After a brief visit we all went to bed hoping to sleep some before the full array of tests scheduled for the next day. I spent that night as I spent part of each night listening to see if Tom was breathing. I touched my husband often just to feel his chest rise and fall. Breathing was an effort for Tom; he slept fitfully and I slept little and lightly.

The drive to the building that housed admissions was between an office building and the pediatric wing of the hospital. A circle drive allowed patients access to the hospital's multiple front doors. The driveway was filled with cars and shuttle buses depositing and picking up patients, families and workers. We had not gotten a wheelchair for Tom at the hotel, but debarking from the shuttle bus he was so weak that we got one when we entered the hospital's foyer. Protesting, Tom got in it, and when he saw the distances he would travel from station to station for his tests, I think he was grateful for it. As a medical professional, Tad was impressed from our initial moments at the admission desk with the organization of the Cleveland Clinic. Tom's itinerary for the day of tests had been carefully planned. People at every level among those we encountered were warm, friendly, helpful, and concerned. Tad had not heard much about *family-centered care* at this point in his medical career, but that was clearly the standard at Cleveland. Early that morning we met Dr. Young, the physician who would become Tom's transplant cardiologist in Cleveland. At the

Cleveland Clinic the patient check-in areas, at least in the cardiology area, were named a letter and a number, thus we met Dr. Young at F 16. This was our first stop after Admissions. As we waited, a young, female physician's assistant called Tom's name. She took a very thorough history before introducing us to Dr. Young. We were not shocked when Dr. Young agreed that the records he had been sent from our cardiologist in Arkansas indicated Tom's heart was in terrible shape and that a transplant was really our only option. With warmth and professionalism the doctor assured us that the Cleveland Clinic would make every effort to do what was best for Tom. The test procedures began with a blood draw, an electrocardiogram, and chest x-rays. None of us remember the order of procedures done the remainder of the day. Things moved smoothly without wasted time between tests, a fact that particularly impressed our son. There was an echocardiogram done, and Tom remembers a treadmill done specifically to measure the utilization of oxygen by his lungs. He walked with a tube in his mouth that measured the gases he exhaled. The only hang up of the day occurred at this test station. The Fellow supervising the test needed the serial or model number of Tom's defibrillator. We did not know it and Tom didn't have a card with that information on it as patients often do. The physician and technician would not proceed with the test without the serial number. Tad made several frantic trips to the telephone trying to reach Dr. Anthony who had been Tom's cardiologist in Arkansas when the device was implanted. Finally Tad got the needed information and the test was completed. I have always wondered if we had not been able to get the information about the defibrillator in Tom's chest would the Fellow have stopped everything and waited, working us into the schedule another day? Tom was so thoroughly evaluated that I think it unlikely that any of the tests would have been skipped. We were moved efficiently from one hospital area to the next. An uncommunicative Fellow who would neither talk with Tom about what he was seeing, nor position Tom so that he could see the screen himself, supervised Tom's ultrasound. My husband, who was accustomed to watching such procedures, was not pleased. One of the most difficult tests of the day for Tom was a CT scan. We had gone down into the basement of the hospital for this one. The waiting room was tiny. The technicians wanted Tom to hold his arms and shoulders a certain way. After a while the pain from holding that position was excruciating. My husband told them he could not continue the test. It was so out of character for Tom to complain. The technicians were not through gathering information so they recruited Tad to hold Tom's arms which they had braced with pillows until they could complete the examination. As the hours passed we did not have time to eat. I was concerned about a drop in Tom's sugar level and how that would affect the tests as well as what it would do to him in his weakened condition. By this time Tom was beyond exhaustion. He sat slumped and silent in his wheelchair. The good people of the Cleveland Clinic were making a great effort to get all Tom's tests done, and the data gathered for evaluation in one day. Our airline ticket home was for the next morning, and it was obvious that Tom needed to get back to the heart failure clinic and to his I.V. medication. When we were in Ohio for Tom's evaluation, approximately forty heart catheterizations were done at the Cleveland Clinic on any given day. The hands on the waiting room clock showed nearly 4:00 p.m. when Tom's name was called, and an attendant wheeled him to the cath lab. He looked so frail as they took him away. Tad hurried to the cafeteria to eat a very late lunch as soon as his father was rolled out of sight. I did not want to leave the waiting room although the attendants said I had plenty of time before Tom's test would be finished. Food was not allowed in the waiting room, but there was a coffee machine. I had overdosed on black coffee; between a bad case of coffee nerves and the stress we were already under I do not think I could have eaten anything. Tad was soon back in the waiting room with me. He and I watched the clock knowing that he had a flight leaving early in the evening for Tennessee. I desperately wanted him in the waiting room when the cardiologist came out to talk to us, not only because he is our son, but also because as a physician he might understand more of the report than I. We waited. The once overcrowded waiting room had several vacant spaces, more as the clock on the wall ticked its way toward 6:00 p.m. Tad explained to a person at the receptionist's desk that he had a plane to catch soon, and that if it was at all possible he would like a report on his father before he had to leave. At last the cardiologist who was doing Tom's arteriogram called Tad to the inner sanctum. I don't know if our son actually went into the cath lab or if the doctor met him somewhere in the rooms beyond where we waited. Dr. Rincon spoke to Tad as a physician to physician courtesy to let him know that Tom was withstanding the test. When our son returned to the waiting room to grab his bags, he tried to reassure me by saying that if Tom could just hang on long enough to get to the Cleveland Clinic as a prospective organ recipient; we would be in good hands. The hospital staff had instilled confidence in our son on both personal and professional levels. With a quick hug Tad was gone to catch a cab and, I hoped, to make his flight. Another hour passed. The waiting room was almost empty because normal business hours had ended. Waiting for a catheterization of Tom's heart to be complete was certainly not a new experience for me, but the hospital and its personnel were new to us both. Time dragged allowing me to focus on how weak Tom had been as they wheeled him away for the cath; how pale; how tired. I began to fear that my husband had coded, or perhaps that he had bled out through the puncture in his groin as he had almost done once before. My fears were taking control. Just then a very courtly, kind, and soft spoken gentleman came into the waiting area. The attendant called my name. The doctor identified me and came directly to the area where I was sitting. Throughout the day, especially after Tad left, I had inched closer and closer to the door to the cath lab. Dr. Rincon did not have far to walk to reach my chair. He sat beside me and holding both my hands in his told me that Tom had come through the procedure just fine; that I would shortly be called back to sit with him; that he had verified Tom's condition, and that we would be hearing from the Clinic. I thanked the doctor for taking time even though it was after hours to talk with me; he acknowledged my thanks; said something about his wife would be waiting dinner, and was gone. In a short while I was allowed into the holding area where Tom was to lie still until the groin puncture from the arteriogram clotted. I thought this meant the six to eight hours it would have taken at home. I did not know how either of us, especially Tom, could hold out. My husband, however, had been introduced to the collagen plug as a stopper for the puncture site. Collagen is a fibrous protein material. It will adhere to tissue and bone in humans and dissolve in a matter of days without harm to the patient. Thanks to this fantastic plug our wait was to be much shorter. Tom was given a snack. The nursing staff was attentive and encouraging. We were among the few people remaining in the holding area since it was late. It was 8:00 p.m. when the nurse checked Tom's collagen plug and we were released. Tom was too weak to walk even if they would have allowed it. I wheeled him to the elevator and to the front of the hospital.

Cleveland Clinic has a really good shuttle system. The small buses run day and night around a campus that covers many city blocks, some of it in an area where one might not feel comfortable walking at night. I got Tom's wheelchair curbside to wait for the next shuttle which was already on its way up the drive. It was cold and windy there on the shores of Lake Erie. Tom was worn out and weak as I helped him from the wheelchair onto the shuttle. His color was bad, and he was frustrated that he was so weak that he needed help boarding the shuttle bus. At the next stop a woman carrying a small Christmas tree boarded the bus. She was excited to have gotten the tree at a bargain. Turning to me Tom asked why she had bought a tree after Christmas. Being oxygen-starved, his thinking was sometimes fuzzy, and for a moment he thought the holidays were past. One of the difficult things for me during this phase of Tom's heart failure was seeing him not always able to think clearly when a sharp mind and his quick wit were such a part of the personality I loved. The bus deposited us at the hotel door where I got another wheelchair and took him upstairs to our room. Determined to get him to eat something I ordered a dinner he ordinarily enjoyed of pasta with chicken and cream sauce but he barely touched it. Although we were exhausted neither of us rested well.

The morning of December 19, we caught a cab to the airport for our flight home. Tom says he remembers the wonderful aroma of cinnamon buns floating through the air from a concession at the terminal. We had not eaten breakfast and as delicious as those smelled, he knew the sugar content would torpedo his system, and in a burst of making responsible food choices we passed them by. We did grab a bite of something, just nothing as enticing as that cinnamon bun. Knowing very little of if, or when, Tom might be accepted into the transplant program at the Cleveland Clinic, we boarded our flight. I remember thinking throughout the trip back to Arkansas that if Tom was not accepted soon, it would be too late. In a letter dictated the day he met Tom, Dr. Young does mention some concern about the number of *sternotomies*, chest openings, Tom had been through. Dr. Young's letter also states that the patient has been told to call him on January 6, after he has the test results, and has discussed the case with Dr. McCarthy, the cardiac transplant surgeon, and the transplant team, as well as with Tom's cardiologist in Arkansas, Dr. Drew.

13

Waiting

We are not good waiters, Tom and I, but that is how Christmas, New Year's, and all of January passed with us waiting. We arrived, energy sapped, back in Arkansas on Friday afternoon which meant that Tom faced a minimum of forty eight more hours with no IV medication for his heart failure. Monday, December 23, he was relieved to be back under the care of Nori and Margie. The clinic notes from that day reflect that he was in atrial fibrillation; his heart rhythm was out of sync. He resumed the five hour drip of the same two medicines he had taken prior to our trip to Cleveland. As at Thanksgiving the specter of this being our last Christmas hung heavy over all of us in spite of our efforts to keep things light, especially in front of our grandchildren. For the first time in his life Tom was unable to go to his mother's home on Christmas morning. Being home for Christmas had been so important to him that the first year we were married he, to my embarrassment, had us knocking on their front door before his parents and much younger sisters were awake! Before this Christmas season spending money was scarce. Things at the business were in rapid decline; people inexperienced in management were in charge; Tom could not focus enough to fully comprehend what was happening. Our income had been severely cut and my husband was on disability. Knowing that it was too expensive for us to maintain, we sold our Suburban. I worried a lot about Christmas gifts that year. I love giving, and start planning well in advance for individualized presents that I hope the recipients will really enjoy. I had neither the time nor the funds in 2002 to do that. I remember making Barbie doll clothes for the two oldest granddaughters, but I have no recollection of what I did for anyone else. I do know that my dad gave us a laptop computer for our trip to Cleveland so I could pay our bills and communicate with the folks at home. I sit here now writing on it.

Christmas Eve and Christmas Day Tom was at home, but on Thursday he went back to the heart failure clinic where he had another visit with Dorothy. Her waiting experience had been different from ours because she received her heart at a center within a day's travel distance from Arkansas. She had been allowed to wear a paging device. Prior arrangements had been made for her to fly to St. Louis by private plane once she received the call that a suitable heart had been found. She continued to pray with and to encourage Tom. He was off for New Year's Eve, and New Year's Day, and then back in the heart failure clinic on January 3, 2003, for his five hour treatment. When Tom called Cleveland on January 6, as he had been instructed to do, there was no news. On January 8, Tom heard from Dr. Young, the Medical Director of the transplant unit. The transplant team needed a CT of Tom's heart in order to complete their evaluation. That was done locally and sent to the Cleveland Clinic. We continued to wait. Margie admonished Tom on his next several visits to the heart failure clinic to continue weighing himself daily. Without enough energy to eat, Tom was losing too much weight, and this was a point of concern.

As difficult as this time was, many good things happened even as we were being tested near to the limits of our endurance. Just before our trip to Cleveland for Tom's evaluation as a transplant candidate, I attended what had become an annual Christmas lunch with old friends, some I've known since college, others not quite so long. Most of us have raised our children together, attended school functions, Scout functions, and various ladies' clubs together, but our greatest common thread is that during those years we were raising our families we were all members of the same church. As time passed, most of us had moved on to other congregations. Missing each other, and not wanting to lose touch, we planned to meet for lunch once a month, usually at a restaurant. At Christmas, however, we met in the home of a particular member for a more festive time. It was from this woman that we had derived, in jest, the name for our group. We were *The Board*; she was actually on a board, and we thought that sounded important enough to get us excused from other demands on our time if we said we had a *board meeting*. In the beginning we had exchanged little gifts at Christmas, but over the years we had decided that it would be more meaningful if we pooled our resources and gave a cash gift to a charity of our choice. Our gift was usually in the range of fifteen to twenty-five dollars each. During the Christmas season that year twenty-five dollars was hard for me to find, but I desperately wanted to be with my friends, and I did not want them to know the full truth of how difficult things were for Tom and me. I saved enough money and went to the board meeting. There must have been twenty of us there for soup, sandwiches and pie; this menu had become a tradition for us. After our meal and some visiting, one of the ladies mentioned that it was time for us to give our gift. Praying that no one upped the ante, I got out my money to add to the rest. Instead of taking my money those precious friends handed me a thousand dollars for *meal money* in Cleveland. As important as the money was, and I don't think they knew the full extent of that, their expression of love was worth so much more. We cried, and hugged, and wished our Merry Christmases smiling through some tears. I drove home overwhelmed by the generosity of *The Board* and with a heart full of gratitude for their love and support. I thanked God for giving us such caring friends and I could not wait to tell Tom. When I did, we both wept.

Friends and family called, dropped by and sent cards to let us know they cared. God was using this time and all of the expressions of love that we received to grow and to reinforce our faith. A friend we had known since college days but didn't see often, called to say that she attended church with a man who had received a heart several years ago at the Cleveland Clinic. She made arrangements for us to meet him and his wife. The four of us got together one afternoon for coffee so we could hear their story. The deterioration of Roy's heart had not been the long journey Tom's had. Roy had suffered a massive coronary attack that had resulted in his being transported to Cleveland almost immediately. He and his wife were warm and encouraging, and their story gave us hope as well as a sense that the Cleveland Clinic was the right choice for Tom. These two new friends brought us a book of scripture, and a hand-held game to help Tom pass the time. Roy and Barbara told us to call them anytime with whatever questions we might have. After exchanging phone numbers, addresses, and e-mail addresses we parted promising to stay in touch. Three of us hugged or shook hands, but our new transplanted friend would not shake hands. He had absorbed all of the Clinic's teaching about the germs spread by infrequently washed hands; rather than risk the germs with a handshake, he touched elbows, an amusing and effective dodge of a very real problem for people with suppressed immune systems. We agreed to meet again, and when we did we found ourselves seated near a group of ladies, who upon hearing snatches of our conversation, realized that Tom was the person their group had been praying for in their church. One of the women introduced herself as a friend of Tom's parents from years past. In our town we were prayed for by people of all denominations; prayers we not only gratefully accepted, but that we coveted. Sometimes people from different congregations sent us their church bulletins with Tom's name on the prayer list or dropped us a note or card to say that they were praying for Tom. We do not underestimate the power of such prayer.

We had been home from Cleveland just over a month. I was worried that they had decided that Tom was not a good risk for the program because of the number of times his chest had been opened. That alone, not his age, or his Type II diabetes, or anything else had merited mention in our discussions with Dr. Young. Tom called a time or two to speak with Renee, the pre-transplant nurse who had been our initial contact at the Clinic. Patient and personable, she always responded that as soon as she knew something, we would know. It was a tense time. Watching someone you love move inexorably toward death is difficult. I was praying for miracles.

Although an unhappy situation in our daughter's life had brought her back to Arkansas, and illness and the loss of a job had kept her here, even this testing time in her life was used for good by God. She became our chief encourager and cheerleader. Even with the responsibility of going to school and caring for her daughter, she stepped in, bolstering us and accepting the responsibility of caring for my father when the call came for us to go to Ohio. As dad had often said, and not in a complimentary way, to me since mom died-*Mary* (meaning my mother) *never cooked anything like this*, so he would say to my daughter although he ate most every bite of what was set before him. Leigh was my mainstay on the home front.

One of the pastors of the church we attended, a woman with a servant's heart, came by to visit and to pray. An associate pastor, on another afternoon, surprised us by ringing the bell. He was a quiet man, a big man. We didn't know him well and were surprised to see him standing at our front door. He asked to come in and visited with us for a while. Most all visitors were careful of staying too long since they could see it was difficult for Tom to maintain enough energy and air to talk for extended periods. As Jeff prepared to leave he handed Tom two thousand dollars from the church's Good Samaritan Fund for our expenses in Cleveland. Never had we expected such a gift. As Jeff prayed we felt humble before God and this good man. Yes, the material support we received was important; it helped provide a feeling of security for the days ahead. The prayer support, however, was primary. Prayer warriors were assaulting the gates of heaven on Tom's behalf. Friends from The Board and a couple of clubs and Bible studies made up a prayer calendar with each friend taking a day of the month to pray specifically for Tom and me. A minister who had been our daughter's pastor when she had lived in North Carolina was now at a church in Italy; he led our international e-mail prayer chain. We believe that even as God chastened and tested us, He was also behind this huge outpouring of love and support for us. We had not earned it; we did not deserve it, but mercifully and graciously it was ours.

The last week in January we got the call. Tom had been accepted as a probable candidate for a heart transplant at the Cleveland Clinic. Official notice of his clearance to be placed on the heart transplant waiting list with a status assigned to him would not come until later. He had his last treatment at the local heart failure clinic January 30. We made preparations for the trip of a lifetime. When that call came, and that word went out among our friends and family, they redoubled their efforts to love and to encourage us bringing muffins for us to snack on as we drove; books to read as we waited in Cleveland, and more cards, some with checks in them. One friend brought me a box of note cards already stamped and ready for me to use. Several people gave us prepaid phone cards to cover our calls home so we could stay in close touch with our support group. Cell phones were now the norm and we had one, but they were not allowed nor did they work in all parts of the hospital. Our supper club signed a down-filled lap throw with their good wishes and gave it to Tom. One of our friends had heard how cold it was in the winter in Cleveland and brought over fleece tunics for me to wear. Kindness piled on top of kindness. Two couples dear to our hearts, devout believers, came to hold their hands on Tom and to pray over him. What strength we gained from being lifted up this way! Finally the night before we left, one long-time friend, a singer, brought us a basket of goodies and a tape she had made especially for us to encourage us on our journey. Our packing was done. The car, a thirteen-year-old Mazda, was loaded. We had been advised by Renee, our liaison with the team in Cleveland to come prepared to stay at least six months. It never occurred to me that I would not stay there with Tom for as long as it took. Given the distress our business was experiencing was that wise? Possibly not, although I believe the fate of the business was already set and anything I could have done would have had minimal effect on the eventual outcome. At any rate there was no question but that Tom was too ill to go alone.

He would be hospitalized upon our arrival. I would be housed in the P Building, more about that later.

On a cold, gray day, February 2, 2003, Tom and I pulled out of our drive with me behind the wheel of the Mazda praying we would not run into snow or slick roads. Every available bit of space in the trunk and back seat was filled with those bits and pieces with which we would try to make Cleveland feel like home for however long it took. Our daughter, granddaughter and my father waved from the carport as we pulled into traffic. Tom's mother and one of his sisters had been by the evening before. Hopeful about the possibilities that could lie ahead; heartsick about the possibility that *might* lie ahead; we continued balancing on our emotional tightrope, dancing tentatively and fearfully on the wire, not always recognizing the safety net of God's love in place beneath us.

14

Arrival

On all of our vacations if we were driving Tom had always pushed for an early start. This trip we did not get away until later in the day. Perhaps that reflects our difficulty in leaving the familiar and facing the unknown. It may have been only that I was slow in getting everything in our small car, and checking it off my list item by item. The first leg of our trip was a boring and familiar one, the highway to Memphis. We needed to stop about every two hours for Tom to walk a bit to keep the circulation in his legs working properly, so stopping in Memphis fit the bill. More importantly, it was the home at that time of our son and his family. I remember that we waited for our grandson and granddaughter to get off the school bus so we could see them. After a quick visit with hugs, kisses, and heartfelt good wishes, we pulled from another driveway leaving more of those we loved waving in the distance. Reluctant to say good-bye, our son led us by a shortcut back to Interstate 40. The three of us lingered over coffee in a small roadside restaurant before Tad turned back to his family and we continued our journey. It was so hard to say goodbye. Tom and I were now alone, something we had never been in all the years of Tom's illness and surgeries. We didn't make it far that first night, only to Jackson, Tennessee. Tom insisted that we share the driving, which troubled me, but I chose not to fight that battle. I was deeply concerned about the weather as we got nearer to our destination. I had limited experience driving on snow, and I knew I did not drive well on ice. I did not want Tom stressed out either by riding with me on slick roads, or by driving on them himself which I knew he would try to do. Tom was worried about our thirteen-year-old automobile. He knew it had a small leak in the radiator hose. Fortunately, it leaked only when the engine was turned off. We carried extra anti-freeze. Tom remembers that February 2 was the day that the space shuttle burned on re-entry. Like many Americans we were stunned and saddened by that horrible accident. Saturday morning dawned very cold but sunny. We took to the road with glad hearts which sounds odd, but in some ways we seemed to have the ability to enjoy this trip together. The enforced togetherness of an enclosed car made us discuss some things we needed to discuss; it allowed us to share some memories that were meaningful, and because we needed to stop so often to stretch our legs, we had to slow down, something neither of us does well. Our budget was tight and fast food was bad for Tom, so we ate a good breakfast and picnicked on foods we had brought from home, some of them goodies from our friends. Picnicking in the winter in a fully loaded car can be a challenge. Certainly there was no getting out and finding a table at the windswept roadside visitors' centers. The sunshine held although there were encroaching clouds. We listened to music when we tired of talking, especially the tape Nancy had sung for us. Occasionally Tom napped when it was my turn to drive

By afternoon we were passing large farms with snow in the furrows of the fields and there was snow along the roadside, but none was falling. We made better time and drove further than we had anticipated being able to do. We passed Cincinnati and picked up the interstate highway we would stay on to Cleveland. Tom and I had agreed that even if it was early when we made it to the other side of Columbus, Ohio we would stop for the day. I remember particularly the name of the little village where we found a motel for our second night on the road; it was Sunbury, Ohio. The name seemed cheerful and quite fitting as we watched a spectacular sunset over the snow-covered farm fields surrounding the motel. After finding a bite to eat we settled in for the night. We probably called home to report our whereabouts and to set my dad's mind at ease. Bless his heart; he still thought of me as his little girl, and he wanted to know I was safe so far from home. Tom and I were developing the habit of praying together each evening, sometimes aloud, and I remember our prayers of gratitude for the good weather and for no problems with the car. We were less than two hundred miles from Cleveland.

Sunday morning, we started the last leg of our journey full of anticipation and some anxiety. We had not driven into Cleveland before.

Finding one's way in a large and unfamiliar city can be a challenge even under the best of circumstances. We probably did not realize at the time how fortunate we were to be having that experience on a Sunday rather than in the midst of rush-hour traffic on a work day. We passed Hopkins Field, the airport into which we had flown for Tom's evaluation in December. We passed the baseball field, and saw ads for the Rock and Roll Hall of Fame, but for the most part that portion of the west side of the city was as depressed looking as it had seemed that evening we viewed it from a cab. Cities don't put their best foot forward along the interstate. Before we reached the city limits, Tom had taken over the wheel of the car. I was the navigator for this final leg of our trip, looking for street signs as he drove. We either passed near or intersected Interstate 90, which set Tom to reminiscing about a trip we had made to Erie, Pennsylvania with Tad and his wife, Laura, for a friend's wedding. Tom had slipped off during the trip and driven to Mentor, Ohio to fly a little ultra-light airplane called the Titan Tornado. He still relished the memory. At last we glimpsed the Cleveland Clinic signs, and then we saw the buildings. We were searching for Euclid Avenue and for the correct parking lot for the P Building where I would be housed. There were one way streets; there was construction but we arrived at the right spot only to find that it was a gated parking lot and we could not enter it. Tom found a friendly guard who raised the gate for the car and pointed us to the correct level for P Building residents to park. I was happy that we could park in a covered area.

We found a place near the walkway to our entry but the door was locked and we could not enter. Within moments some people came out, and Tom was able to go in. He still had to find the correct elevator and pick up the key to our third floor room. I waited with the car after I snagged an empty wheelchair from inside the building to use as a luggage cart. As I waited for Tom to return I took from our trunk boxes of food, dishes, books, and of course, the laptop that would be our lifeline to Arkansas. The parking area for the transplant patients and their families was near one of the designated smoking areas for hospital employees and guests. The cold air reeked of smoke and was hazy. I was not pleased that each time my husband came back to the car he would have to walk through that. Tom returned with room keys and a small manila envelope of instructions for our stay. As determined as he was to help carry things into the building, I was more determined that he would not. I pushed the fully loaded wheelchair and he wielded the card key to get us into the building. With six months worth of supplies, I had several trips to make. When at last it was all in the room and, if not stored in its final space, it was at least where we would not trip over it, we rested. My new home was very much like a college dormitory room, or perhaps like a room one might find in an older motel. There were two full-size beds, a couple of chairs and a table, a dresser and mirror, a space for hanging clothes and a television. Each room had its own bath complete with a tub and an overhead shower. While everything wasn't new, it was all very clean and quite comfortable. Only when you went into the bathroom did you get a sense of being a part of a hospital because there was an emergency cord attached to the wall for patients needing assistance. The P Building housed persons waiting for transplants and those recuperating from transplant surgeries as well as their families. Our view was another section of the hospital complex, the pediatric wing with its cheerfully painted windows; across the street was the cafeteria. We had our dinner there after exploring the admissions area of the hospital where Tom would register as a patient the following morning. The P Building was quite a distance from all of these things. It was, however, all under the same roof, and I was excited to be where I would not have to drive or catch a bus to the hospital each day in a cold and unfamiliar city. Had I not been able to live in the P Building, there were people in the city who opened their homes to transplant families for a very small fee. The P Building also had a small charge. We could not have afforded for me to stay in a hotel, and because there were not ordinarily private rooms on the transplant floor, staying in the room with Tom was not an option. I would have been forced to return home leaving him to wait alone.

Tom was scheduled for more tests Monday morning. We rose early and dressed. He was not to eat and I wasn't hungry. I did walk down to the communal kitchen and found that some early riser had already made a pot of coffee. I grabbed a paper cup of coffee and met Tom at the elevator. We had not yet learned our way around the hospital but we knew we had to get from Building P to Building H for Tom to register for admission at Desk 10. We took an elevator to the second floor where we walked through an immense waiting area. We did not know it, but this was the surgery waiting area where I would later wait for Tom to receive his new heart. After crossing this room, we walked down a long corridor past a pediatric section of the Clinic, and more waiting rooms, then up an intersecting hall lined with offices and research rooms, before we finally reached the elevator that would take us to the first floor of the H Building. Perhaps it was less than a quarter mile distance, but I think not. Once on the ground floor we were able to find Desk 10 and sign Tom in. There were, of course, the usual questions to be answered and cards to be copied. When that was completed the registrar told us to take a seat until we heard Tom's name called. Renee had said that she would meet us at H 10 Monday morning to introduce Tom to what he could expect. We found seats in this vast combination foyer and waiting area, and waited and waited. No one came. I'm sure we did not wait as long as it seemed we did. We probably, since it is Tom's habit, arrived early, and since we were already anxious, the waiting only made us more so. At last Tom's name was called and we were taken to the M Building where nurses put us in a private room, brought Tom some hospital pajamas, told him to undress and get into them, and that they would return to get a history. We had not expected a private room and were pretty excited. We were wondering when we would get to meet Renee but assumed that she had been delayed. Tom was almost into the pajamas, and I was stashing his street clothes in a bag when the nurses reappeared telling him to stop undressing and to put on his clothes again. They were somewhat shamefaced, but Tom had been mistaken for someone else with a similar name, and taken to the wrong area of the hospital. Renee had been searching for him for thirty minutes. She and her assistant entered, making multiple apologies for temporarily losing us. Tom was, she said, going to be in the intensive care unit, not the M Building. It had not occurred either to Tom or to me that he would go immediately to ICU in Cleveland. After all, his heart failure treatment at home even after it became daily, had been as an outpatient.

In ICU Tom was given a hospital gown, not the comfy pajamas he had almost worn in Building M, and I was told that the visiting hours were sparse and strictly observed. Then I was sent to a tiny waiting room where I spent most of the day, not too sure I could find my way back to the P Building, or that if I found my way back anyone would know where to find me if Tom needed me. Meanwhile, once again confined to a windowless coronary cubicle, Tom was rebelling against the rules. He was determined that I would be allowed to see him more often than the rules allowed; his male nurse was equally as determined that I would see my husband at the stated visiting hours. Eventually a truce was called and Tom was told that for those patients who proved cooperative, allowances in visiting privileges might be made. Tom was still on all of the oral medication he had been taking in Little Rock, but at this point he had no IV's. He was scheduled for more tests to ascertain his suitability to be placed on the transplant list. The first test was an extremely thorough dental examination. Unlike the earlier evaluation tests done in December when he had gone to many different areas of the hospital, these tests were all done in the intensive care unit with the specialists and their equipment coming to him. Following the dental exam were more x-rays, one I think to check his gallbladder again to see if the pebble-size stones they had noted in December had traveled. They had not. When at last I was called back for visiting hours I found Tom's nurse to be a reasonable young man who liked duck hunting. When he learned we were from Arkansas he wanted to know all about the duck hunting in our state. I remember that I got someone to e-mail me a copy of one of the recipes for duck from our local cookbook for him. While I was in the room with Tom one of the cardiology Fellows, a young Irishman from Dublin, came in to examine my husband. Tom recalls that the Fellow was quite vocal about one of the prescriptions Dr. Drew had Tom on to relieve the load on his heart-he did not like it. He also was not sure that he thought Tom's condition warranted his waiting in Cleveland; he thought perhaps Tom would do just as well to wait at home. That frightened me. I could just see us being told to return to Arkansas to wait now that we were in Cleveland with all our things. What if we couldn't get back when we needed to? My mind ran away with fears, and I did not much like this young Irishman I thought. Sometime after I visited Tom, he remembers that Dr. Young, his transplant cardiologist came by with the usual gaggle of residents and Fellows in tow. Tom was to have a colonoscopy the next morning, and Dr. Young explained that he would be prepped that night, and that the specialist and the equipment for the test would be brought to him in the ICU the next morning. Tom remembers being hooked to so many wires that he could not move to the bedside commode without help all that night. Each ICU patient had an assigned nurse sitting just outside his area. Of course with the medicine he was taking that night, Tom slept very little. Sometime very late he heard a code called and he could hear his nurse as well as others scramble to assist. He remembers thinking that someone had died. At last he slept fitfully.

Back in the P Building, I took some soup I had brought from home down to the kitchen to heat and ate it in my room. I had intended to talk with the concierge that day about how they expected payment for my room, but we had left the building before she came to her office and I had returned so late that she was already gone for the day. I saw a few people wandering our hall, some friendly, some not so much. I locked my door, sat on the bed and tried to process my thoughts about the events of the day before I e-mailed our daughter, our son, and family and friends back home.

Tom remembers that this colonoscopy was remarkable because he was not put to sleep but rather was given something to make him relax that made him extremely talkative. He managed to position himself so that he could watch the screen with the physician. When the tests were completed our Irish Fellow made rounds and again commented that he really thought Tom might wait at home. When I heard that a second time I decided to find out if that was Dr. Young's plan, so when he came through later I asked him. He said no, Tom would not go so far away as Arkansas to wait for a heart and while he did not yet have status on the organ transplant list, he was to be moved to H 11, the heart floor, and IV therapy for heart failure would be begun again but with a different medication than had been used in Arkansas. Dr. Young started Tom on a milrinone infusion twenty-four hours a day, seven days a week. Other medication changes were made as well. Tom spent one more night in ICU before moving.

15

Life on H 11

On the third morning of our life as citizens of the Cleveland Clinic, Tom graduated from the intensive care unit to the transplant floor. It was another step in the right direction, and we were both excited to be moving. His first room had no other patient in it, but the nurses told him not to get accustomed to that luxury because private rooms were not the norm. I only know of two patients who had private rooms during our entire stay; one was a lung transplant patient who was not doing well, and one was a local physician who had suffered through two consecutive transplants when the first one failed. The Clinic did have, on another floor, private rooms or suites for the many international dignitaries who choose to be treated there. I am certain that our care equaled theirs in every way. A new heart transplant wing has since been added to the hospital; so much has changed. Without a roommate there was no question but that Tom got the bed by the window. We were told that as the length of stay increased roommates were often switched from one side of the room to the other so each had an opportunity to enjoy the view. The view was spectacular. We not only got a bird's eye view of the hospital campus, at least part of it, and the surrounding neighborhood, but we could clearly see Lake Erie in the distance. The lake was frozen for as far out as we could see, but it must have not frozen over completely that winter. The city of Cleveland received 108 inches of snow the winter of 2002-2003. The all time record was 111 inches. The natives told us that when Lake Erie was entirely frozen, less snow fell. So much snow, the frozen Great Lake; it was all a novelty to us. It also intensified my thankfulness for the P Building. On H 11 there were not set visiting hours so I was able to spend most of my time with Tom. The rooms were not large, but there were recliners, and each room had its own bath. I felt when we reached the eleventh floor that we were safe from being sent back to Arkansas to wait. Tom's IV to reduce the load on his heart was started and although the move had tired him, he immediately felt some relief from that. At some point during the day two central venous lines were put in Tom, one in his right chest and one in his neck, to avoid multiple needle sticks each day. His hands and arms where the milrinone was infused had become increasingly more difficult to stick as his time on intravenous therapy lengthened. The line in his chest, something called a Swan-Ganz catheter, gave the doctors direct access to the pulmonary artery allowing multiple daily measurements of Tom's cardiac output and related information. The line in his neck went to his jugular vein, a direct venous route to the heart, from which the physicians also drew several small vials of blood each day. When Tom's lunch tray arrived I made the quarter-mile hike back to the P Building to prepare a bite for myself and to pick up the laptop and various other things to help us settle into our new *home*. It is odd how your horizons narrow and you settle into a routine as you wait for things to happen over which you have no control. I have wondered if this is how people who are confined feel, and if they also cope by creating *busyness*, and ways to make the time go by. Tom was exhausted and spent the rest of that first day on H 11 in his bed. Hooked to IV's and still in heart failure there was little exercise that he could, or should do. He was encouraged to walk the hall a couple of times a day as he felt like doing it, and that became part of our routine. At either end of the hall were solariums where he could stop to rest, enjoying the change of scene and the terrific view of Lake Erie. Each day I would bring the laptop to his room so that he could play computer games, but he soon found that he had difficulty concentrating on those for any length of time. I brought him books and letters from friends and family, reports of phone calls and e-mails from Arkansas. I read to him, and we read the Bible together. One of the first things I brought to his room was the lap throw our supper club friends had signed with good wishes and sent along with us. It seemed Tom was always cold and the throw warmed both body and spirit. My own spirit warmer was a pin given me by a friend before we left Little Rock. It was a little silver and gold wheelbarrow full of red hearts. I wore it every day we were in Cleveland.

Tom got his first roommate on H 11 in the middle of his first night. Like all but one of those with whom he shared a room, this was a nice gentleman with a kind and thoughtful family. He was from Chillicothe, Ohio, a little older than Tom and very frightened. He was not a transplant candidate but had been transferred to Cleveland Clinic for other reasons. He was scheduled for tests and possible surgery. His adult daughters introduced us to what became our special treat in Cleveland, a caramel, warm, apple cider concoction from the Starbuck's located in the hospital's cafeteria. This gentleman's friends who visited introduced us to a tradition new to us when they stood beside their friend's hospital bed and prayed for him; they all prayed at once, each his own prayer. God's hearing, we decided, was fine tuned to hear His children however and wherever they cried out to Him. Such group prayers were not uncommon in the succession of roommates Tom had. One thing did seem strange, to me at least, not once in the two months we were at the Cleveland Clinic did a hospital chaplain visit Tom's room. I am sure one would have if we had requested a visit, but coming from the Bible belt where a visit from the chaplain, and in our hospital, a nun, was as routine as the daily visit from your physician, it seemed odd. There was a beautiful chapel on the hospital's first floor; again it was unlike the one at home in that it was sometimes locked. I took my quiet time with God in my home in the P Building. One of the television channels available late at night featured a meditation-relaxation program with beautiful photography and soothing music. Most nights I tuned that in as I read my Bible, prayed and tried to sleep.

Our days assumed a pattern on H 11. Rising fairly early I would make my breakfast, and take the hike through the hospital to Tom's room where I would stay until his lunch came. We would walk to a solarium when Tom felt able, perhaps put a piece or two in whatever jigsaw puzzle the community had working at the time, and return to the room. We looked forward to visits from members of a group called *Mended Hearts*. Not all of them were transplant patients, but all had been through heart surgery, and they volunteered their time as encouragers for hospital patients. They were great, but sadly, I think their activities have been curtailed by the HIPPA laws that have since been passed. Tom and I clicked with one particular member of this group and his wife. Paul and Ruby were from the area; they were retired; they were dedicated Christians who felt that Paul had been saved by his transplant to serve others. We looked forward to their visits and their prayers. Paul was about fifteen months out from his transplant and was doing well. Like most of the heart patients we met in Cleveland, his problems with his heart were not the result of a long illness, but rather they were the result of a fast moving virus that weakened and debilitated his heart. His story was unique. Paul, who was the minister of a very small suburban congregation, had been a patient of the Cleveland Clinic with a group of about a dozen men of all ages and backgrounds. As residents of the eleventh floor they became a walking fraternity, helping each other exercise, and bolstering each others' spirits. One by one each man received a new heart until only Paul remained waiting. During that time Paul had been prepared for transplant surgery nine times; a time or two he had even been taken to the operating room. Each time some problem with the donated organ prevented Paul from being transplanted. I cannot imagine going to the brink of a new chance at life nine times and being turned back each time. I think Paul would say that only through his faith in God did he find the courage to keep presenting himself as a transplant candidate. Paul shared with us that he believed his long wait and many false starts toward surgery were part of God's plan to allow him to minister to that group of men, some of whom were not believers. Ruby and Paul never left without praying with us and for us. They insisted that when the call came for Tom to receive a heart I should call them regardless of the hour, and that they would be with me. I did, and they were as good as their word. This godly couple stayed in touch even after we left Cleveland, often meeting Tom at the airport when he returned for tests. They were tremendous encouragers. As time went by the regular nurses on H 11 became our friends, stopping by as time allowed for brief chats. I do not think we had a nurse the entire time we were in Cleveland who did not excel at her job. We loved Karen, a bouncy young nurse from Toledo whose wit and ready smile reminded us of our daughter at home, although they bore no physical resemblance. There was a much older nurse, not an RN, who rode the bus in each evening for her shift. She was Romanian and always called Tom *Sveetie*. The nursing staffs as well as the Cardiology Fellows truly were an international group, a new and interesting experience for us. As the number one heart transplant center in the world the Cleveland Clinic attracted staff, students, and patients from around the globe. During the day Tom was often visited by the Heart Failure Research Coordinator to see if he qualified for various studies. Perhaps the person we grew closest to was our calm, quiet, and efficient transplant social worker, Kay. In spite of a huge patient load she missed very few days stopping by Tom's room to check up on our physical and emotional well-being. Kay was a person we found easy to confide in, the sort of friend you felt you had known all your life. She, better than anyone in Cleveland, understood the financial cloud we were under and the stress it generated. We met Jennifer, Dr. Young's specialty nurse, who with her sunny smile brightened our gray days. Of course it was rare for Tom not to see one of the transplant cardiologists each day with the requisite group of Fellows and residents dutifully following along.

When Tom's lunch came I usually walked back to the P Building for a cup of soup or a sandwich made from my store of canned tuna brought from Arkansas. Sometimes Tom slept awhile after lunch so I used that time to wash clothes, pay bills via the computer, write e-mails, and get to know my neighbors. They were a varied group; not all heart transplant families or candidates, all ages, and from many different areas of the country-more about them later. On occasion I used this time to walk to a nearby drugstore for supplies. There was no other shop near enough for walking, and I did not want to drive. I feared getting lost, or losing control of our car on the wintry streets, and I did not want to lose my covered parking space. I was not prepared for the bitterly cold wind that blew in from Lake Erie. Foolishly making my first walk to the pharmacy without gloves, my fingers were totally numb by the time I walked the three or four blocks back to the hospital. Mid afternoon I would return to Tom's room prepared most days to remain with him until eleven at night. Much of the time he slept or listened to music or we both read. When my husband slept I walked the halls, learning my way around our neighborhood.

Obviously with its number one rating the Cleveland Clinic does many things very well in its cardiology program. The one thing that impressed Tom and me most was their team approach to keeping patients and their families involved in the process of learning about and tending to the patient's care. One afternoon a week was devoted to a class. All who were able to attend were invited. It was held in a conference room on the eleventh floor. The classes were taught by the hospital physicians and department heads and covered every area of interest to a prospective transplant patient. The patients filed in, some of them with their heart assist machines thumping away-usually out of sync, so that when one thumped the other did not, like a group of drummers each following his own beat. Most of the patients were happy to be there to learn or to pass the time; a few were not. We had classes in endocrinology for patients who, like Tom, were diabetic. There was a pharmacology class to introduce patients and families to what could be a dizzying array of transplant drugs, the precise way in which they were to be taken, and their side-effects. There was a great class on some of the problems faced by transplant patients taught by Dr. Taylor, another of the cardiologists. There was a class presented by one of the dieticians. That one was a repeat for us since a similar class had been offered by our hospital in Arkansas. Perhaps the most entertaining, as well as one of the most informative classes was taught by a physician from the Department of Infectious Disease. He was a great speaker who brought home to us all the importance of protecting the compromised immune systems of transplant recipients from infection. He stressed and stressed hand cleanliness and then made us all laugh by admitting that making rounds he often wrote on his own hands, holding his ball-point stained palms up for us to see. It was definitely *do as I say, not do as I do.* All these classes included a question and answer session, and written material for patient and family to study at their leisure. Each speaker gave us a business card with numbers for contacting him if we had more questions. The classes were free and available as often as anyone wanted to repeat them during his wait for a heart.

Most evenings when I heard the porter begin to deliver meals to the patients on Tom's hall I would run down to the cafeteria to buy my one non-Arkansas-purchased meal of the day. Cleveland's hospital food was no better or no worse than that in Arkansas. Hospital food is hospital food. At least in Cleveland they never brought Tom that same piece of rubbery chicken he insisted he had been served for the past twenty years at home! When we had been at the clinic a while, one of the dietitians visited Tom and told me that I could order my dinner to be delivered with Tom's and put it on my P Building tab. After checking my budget, I did that some evenings. We learned that if Tom were hospitalized long enough to become so bored with the food that he did not eat well, we would be offered what was called the Middle Eastern menu as a change. The Clinic saw a great many patients from that part of the world and did their best to observe those dietary laws and habits as well as those more familiar in the western world. As fans of hummus and tabouli, we were excited.

We continued to be concerned about our failing business and our finances. We talked very little about it. I stayed in touch with the plant by e-mail and filtered what I relayed to Tom. There was no good news. At some point we heard from Renee that Tom was on the transplant list but that he was not being considered as someone critical enough to be given a number one status. Within about forty eight hours of learning that Tom was on the list, he developed a sinus infection, which caused his name to be removed from the transplant list. He was started on antibiotics and although we were assured that this was just a bump in the road, it was the low point of our time in Cleveland. As long as Tom had the infection, great pains were taken to have him turn away from the port in his jugular vein when the bandage was removed for a blood draw. It was imperative that he not breathe into an area that led directly to his heart. He ran the risk of introducing the bad bacteria in his sinuses into his heart. February 11, Tom received written notification that he had been placed on the heart transplant waiting list as a status one patient. He would get the next available heart that was a good match for him. It seemed the wait from our arrival at the Clinic until Tom was notified that he was a status one was much longer than it actually was. We celebrated by decorating his window with a string of red foil hearts I had purchased before leaving home. We had already taped drawings from grandchildren and funny cards from friends in spots strategically chosen to generate a smile.

Tom got another new roommate with a family that we enjoyed. This patient also was not a transplant candidate. He was a large man, older than Tom, and his claim to fame was that he grew the largest pumpkins in Ohio. They had won many prizes, and people from all over the United States wrote for seeds from his pumpkins. One of his sons shared a story about a gigantic pumpkin starting to rot; the stench was overwhelming, but the mega-gourd could not be moved until several men managed to load it onto a trailer to be hauled away. We laughed so hard about this pumpkin that sounded like something from an old science fiction movie. When this big family all gathered around their dad I usually went to a solarium to give them space. When Tom was strong enough he walked with me. As Tom's stay on the eleventh floor lengthened we came to know several other patients, and their families as well as hospital personnel. Everyone from the cafeteria porter, to the various Fellows, to the maids who kept the room clean, we knew on sight if not by name. All sharing the same environment, and with many of us focused on the same desired end, we formed an odd but effective brotherhood. Kay, our transplant social worker, was responsible, along with volunteers from the Cleveland area, for organizing a monthly dinner for transplant patients. We were in Ohio only long enough to attend a couple of these. They were great morale boosters. Patients waiting for hearts, those who were recuperating from transplant surgery and others who were several weeks, months or years along gathered with their families to be encouraged by shared stories, and to enjoy the food and fellowship. The youngest attendee at one of our dinners was a child of about seven or eight who was awaiting a transplant. Most diners were adults. This function was held after hours in the Physicians' Dining Room. The stories shared were remarkable for the courage and humility of those who told them. It was impossible in this group to feel alone, or as if you had been especially singled out by God for difficulties. Regardless of the problems you faced, your neighbor had probably faced more. At the first dinner Tom and I were seated next to a couple somewhat younger than ourselves. The husband had been the heart patient and was blind. As we visited during our meal we learned that he had suffered a severe heart attack while exercising. During his transplant surgery Terry had suffered a stroke that had cost him his sight. They were making adjustments to their home to compensate for his sight loss; they were planning a family wedding, and getting on with their lives. I found their attitude amazing, and hoped I could approach their bravery should things go awry for us.

With the exception of the day Tom received a new heart and the day we got to go home, the most exciting day we had in Cleveland was Valentine's Day, February 14. After dinner I was visiting with Tom in his room when the phone rang. People were so great about calling us from home that it was not unusual to hear the voice of our good friend Nancy, but what she said was a tremendous surprise. She and Jim had been in Connecticut visiting their daughter and her family and were traveling by car back to Arkansas. One of their granddaughters was with them and if we could tell them how to find the hospital they were coming by for a visit as soon as they ate a bite of dinner. Tom and I were stunned and overjoyed. Company from home! Wow! What a mood lifter their visit was. The thought that friends loved us enough to go out of their way on a cold and snowy night to find directions through an unfamiliar city to visit us was stunning. Even their teen-age granddaughter seemed to be happy to see Tom although we had never met her. The visit was brief; Tom was both emotional and tired, but those few minutes with friends from home were priceless. I walked down the hall with Nancy, Jim, and Anne after they said their good-byes to Tom. It was so hard to see them get on the elevator and to lose that link with home. When the elevator door closed I had a lump in my throat and tears in my eyes, but we could not have had a better Valentine gift than their surprise visit.

In this world of six degrees of separation, one of Arkansas' Congressmen was also a patient at the Cleveland Clinic during our stay there. His fiancée had been one of the associate pastors of a church we attended. In that role she had visited Tom after his fifth surgery in Little Rock. She looked us up at the Clinic and the four of us visited briefly a couple of times. The Congressman recuperated and went home long before Tom, but before she left with him, our former pastor made arrangements for the minister of a church in nearby Cleveland Heights to meet us. Reverend Dan visited several times and some of his parishioners often called to check on us and to offer their services for shopping. Most meaningful was the fact that Reverend Dan brought us Communion. Sharing the Lord's Supper composed of Reverend Dan's home-made bread and some grape juice never meant more to us than it did in that situation. We hoped to visit Reverend Dan's church on our Easter in Cleveland, but we were back in Arkansas by Easter and Tom's immune system was still too fragile for us to brave the crowd at church.

16

Life in the P Building

Each time I retraced my steps through the hospital's maze of hallways and returned to the P Building, I entered a world Tom did not know. The P Building was a microcosm of any community. We were Caucasian, African-American, and Indian; we were young, middle-aged and older; we were families and singles, male and female. We were bound together by our need when we had nothing else in common.

The majordomo of the P Building was Rose, a statuesque African-American lady with a flair for fashion. Rose ran a tight ship, and worked at hiding a heart of gold. She collected the rent, enforced the house rules, oversaw the housecleaning staff, and on occasion offered a shoulder to cry on. Her wrath was fierce, and her hugs were all enveloping. Rose was the heart and soul of the kingdom she surveyed. The P Building is used for other purposes now. Transplant families are housed on a floor of one of the older hotels on the hospital campus. The rooms are more spacious, the facilities newer, and Rose oversees it all with the same vigor. I cannot help being nostalgic, though, for the closer quarters of the P that demanded interaction, and encouraged the forming of friendships. The population of the P was in constant flux as patients recovered and returned home, or as happened on occasion, a patient passed away and the family left grieving and with hope dashed. Sometimes if space was available, former patients returning for tests and periodic checkups were housed in the P. Tom and I were to stay at the P in this capacity often in the ensuing years. Not all the residents were there because of heart-related problems. The first residents of the P that I met were a young husband and wife, and their children from West Virginia. The husband had received a bone marrow transplant, and was almost ready to go home. Their children were weekend visitors. There was a woman from Michigan whose husband had received a lung transplant. At the end of the hall occupying two rooms was a young family, mother, father, and two children. The father, also named Tom, had received both a kidney and a lung at different times during his battle with cystic fibrosis, with the kidney being the most recent transplant. We continue to exchange e-mail, enjoying pictures of their growing children. Their path has been an arduous one, full of many more ups and downs than ours, but their faith is amazing, and they persist. Tom has recently celebrated his seventeenth year as a successful lung transplant recipient. I remember one older man who was all alone. He was quiet, always seeming to hover on the fringes of any conversation. He was almost ready to return to his home following his heart transplant. I wondered if he would have anybody to encourage him at home, or would he still be alone. I could not help but wonder if I had to leave Tom in Cleveland would he appear so isolated and fragile. We ran into each other in the halls, in the tiny communal kitchen, in the lounge where there was a computer terminal and games. Some of us passed by closed and wanting no company, and others of us shared our stories and our fears, and became an unlikely support system for each other. I recall making friends with another wife. She had lived in the United States for many years but she was originally from India. As we explored each other's backgrounds forming our temporary connection, she shared that hers had been an arranged marriage. Unfamiliar with that custom, I soon learned that our marriages, and our feelings for our husbands were more similar than not. Often I was in the P Building only at night to do laundry, catch up on e-mails and phone calls, pay bills, and try to sleep. I looked forward to the calls from our daughter and my dad as well as from our son and his family. I am sure Leigh and Dad put up a good front to buoy my spirits, but it sounded as if they were working together and handling things at home very well. Dad came up from the little house for dinner most nights, even when, Leigh laughingly remembers, she served him frozen taquitos, a new and not-much liked addition to his palate. Leigh was doing well in school in spite of the added stress. Dad stayed with her in the evening until she got her daughter to bed and the dogs settled in for the night before returning to his home down the hill to sleep. Friends were filling in with meals-Nancy's beer bread and chicken noodle soup, Jan's chicken enchiladas, gift certificates from caterers. Our close friends treated Leigh like their own daughter, calling her often to chat, and to check her progress in school as well as our condition in Cleveland. One of my friends often included our granddaughter in outings to plays, playgrounds and movies that she had planned for her own grandchildren. One couple babysat when needed, giving rise to a rumor that Charles actually played dress-up in fancy hats and jewelry one time with our granddaughter. These were and are amazing friends. Everyone should be so blessed. The supper club and the Bible study friends continued their prayers for us. We always knew from the calendar they had prepared for us who was praying and on what day. Often they e-mailed or called on that day to encourage, or to ask if there was a specific prayer we needed sent to God. Cards and checks continued to be in the mail I would pick up each day in Rose's office. Usually the note on the check said something about the sender wanting us to have this since they couldn't be with us to buy our dinner. The generosity of our friends was humbling. Perhaps they were more aware of my limited budget than I know. Whether they fully understood our situation or didn't, they gave us undeserved love, and a great picture of God's love for us. One friend sent me a weekly newspaper from home and always called on a Sunday night. I don't know how Joy knew that Sunday night was the hardest one for me-maybe she didn't, but her calls were a welcome burst of sunshine during a gloomy time.

Other than Paul and Ruby, the couple we came to know best in Cleveland was Bill and Edna. Bill and Edna were from Ohio, somewhere close to our age, and if anything, Bill needed a heart worse than Tom. He was attached to one of those thumping Left Ventricular Assist Devices. It allowed him to live in the P Building rather than being hospitalized full time like Tom. He could be seen walking the hall with his machine in a wheelchair he pushed along in front of him. Bill was a feisty sort of guy. Tom met him in one of our classes, but I lived just up the hall from Edna and Bill. Often their door was open, welcoming company for Bill, who chaffed at his enforced inactivity. Edna was frequently out shopping which I wondered about until I heard their story. As they were traveling to Cleveland for Bill to be hospitalized to await a heart, their home had burned. Because Bill collected black powder rifles, the house actually exploded once the fire took hold, killing their pet cat, and burning most of their possessions. They had received news that their insurance would help them start over so Edna was trying to find furnishings for the mobile home they would live in while their house was rebuilt. She and one of her daughters also made several trips back to the ruins to try to salvage photographs, or any mementos of Edna's and Bill's former life together. Bill received his heart about ten days before Tom. As luck would have it, Edna was out picking up supplies when Bill got the call. I had just come from Tom's room back to the P to do some chores. I think I had grabbed a load of clothes and was headed to the laundry room when I saw Bill pushing his LVAD in its wheelchair down the hall toward the elevator. He was obviously in a great hurry, and somewhat agitated. I stepped into the hallway and asked him what was going on, and he told me that he had gotten the call and he couldn't wait until Edna got back to go. I dropped my laundry back on the floor of our room and locked the door. I told Bill to get in his wheelchair and hold on to his LVAD, and I had the privilege of pushing him to the door of the surgery suite where the transplant team met him and whisked him away. I think Edna was back at the P about the time I got back to our floor so she was there in time to be with Bill as soon as they would allow her in after the surgery. Getting to have even this tiny part in Bill's success story impacted my life in a huge way. Later as Tom and Bill both recuperated in the P, the four of us decided we wanted to do something to make a difference in the lives of the residents of the P Building, and we wanted to do it to honor our social worker, Kay. None of us were wealthy people but dimes make dollars and dollars make tens. With that in mind we set up a fund to buy recliners for each room in the P. So many of the residents found it difficult to sleep in a bed that we felt this would be a fine addition. We worked with the Cleveland Clinic Foundation in preparing a blurb about our idea for the website. The Foundation was able to find a good price from one of their suppliers, and eventually there were recliners for every room. I am happy to say that those were moved to the transplant families' new quarters when the P was closed.

17

T Day

Tuesday, March 4, 2003, Tom and I had been living in Cleveland for one month. Sometimes it was hard to remain hopeful, but we worked at staying positive. As the day wound to a close we ate dinner together in Tom's room. I think we said our good-nights a little early since Tom's roommate had several family members visiting, and the room was crowded. It was probably not quite nine o'clock as I took one elevator to the first floor, walked through the emptying hospital to another elevator, and went to my third floor room. As usual I enjoyed the many paintings displayed in the halls of the Cleveland Clinic. The more public hallways displayed wonderful, original artwork. My favorite piece was one I walked past daily, a sculpture of a little girl. She resembled one of our granddaughters; I named her Hannah. Reaching my room in the P, I called Tom to tell him I was in for the night. He responded that his roommate's family was gone, and since that gentleman was peacefully asleep and snoring loudly, Tom was putting on his earphones. He planned to listen to some soft music until he slept. I told him that as soon as I e-mailed home and did a couple of chores that I would be going to bed as well. It was my habit to lay out my clothes for the next day on the extra bed in the room in case Tom received a heart in the middle of the night, and I was called to go to his room. I also had taken to wearing my contact lens most nights since I am too nearsighted to see without them, and I wanted to be ready to go in a hurry if called. I set my alarm for 6:30 the next morning and fell into a fitful sleep. I am not sure why I bothered to set my alarm since the garbage truck servicing the hospital cafeteria across the street usually woke me up long before the alarm went off. At 12:46 Tom, still wearing his headphones and sleeping soundly, felt a tug on his toe. He awoke immediately, pulling the headphones from his ears so he could hear what the three nurses standing at the foot of his bed and smiling broadly were saying. One of them, a beautiful young woman who had come from Africa to work and study at the Cleveland Clinic, said to Tom in her musically accented voice that the transplant team had a heart they thought might be a match for him. The nurses instructed him to call me, but they warned him not to get too excited in case this was a dry run and no match. I think I was out of my bed with the first ring of the phone. When I heard Tom say we might have a heart it was impossible to contain my excitement in spite of the cautionary words of the nurses relayed by Tom. Even knowing Paul's story of nine dry runs I threw on my clothes, grateful that I had laid them out. Tom swears he did not know I could move as fast as I did to reach his room that night. Empty hospital halls are full of shadows and can be a bit spooky late at night, but I covered that quarter mile in record time. I'm sure I would have run over anything or anyone who stepped into my path. We called our daughter and our son. We may have called Tom's mother. I think we left that call and the one to Tom's sisters, my dad and our friends for Leigh to handle. I know that Leigh called Linda, the friend one who had often passed herself off to hospital authorities as Tom's sister. She had asked to be called regardless of the hour saying that she would drive to our home to wait with Leigh during her dad's surgery. Leigh thanked her but declined the offer. Instead she sat in Tom's recliner alone in our den, praying and meditating until we called with more news. Tad shared the news with his wife, Laura, and then went into his den to pray. He remembers that he could not stop crying.

Tom and I were speechless and sat smiling at each other and holding hands. I am sure our minds were whirling even if our tongues were silent. We did, when we got our emotions under control and found our voices, pray together. In a short while Tom's nurses returned, and all three of them escorted us, with Tom on a gurney, to the second floor where the operating suites were located. We were turned over to a different set of nurses there. After placing us in a small, brightly lit examining room they left us alone to wait. I don't know how long we waited, not too long, when a very large doctor came into the room. After introducing himself, he was another of our international team, an Egyptian, as the anesthesiologist who would be putting Tom to sleep, he checked the veins in Tom's arms, and did some preparation of sites. Handling Tom with a gentleness that belied his size, he patted my husband's arm incongruously calling him *Dearie*, and was gone. Tom told me that he was at peace; whatever the outcome of this surgery, one way or another he would be going home. Tom says that it was as if the Lord was finally getting the message through to him that He was in charge. Tom had to admit that there was nothing he could do to help himself; he could go forward in complete faith, or he could fight it. At last it seemed to him that there would be no profit in fighting. In the sterile room, under a very bright light Tom smiled and drifted off to sleep. I alternately dozed and prayed as I sat by the gurney and held Tom's hand. Our anesthesiologist was in and out several times. At some point he started a saline drip in Tom's arm. By 5:00 a.m. Tom was still sleeping peacefully and I had decided that this might be a dry run. We got word around eight Wednesday morning, March 5, 2003-*Ash Wednesday*-that the heart had been checked and cross checked for matches with Tom, and that it was now at The Cleveland Clinic. The Heart Surgery Fellow came through the door dressed in the white slacks and shirt that was the uniform of these young doctors. He told us that it was time. Just like that-it was time. My own heart plummeted to my toes, soared, and almost stopped as I rose from the chair where I had spent the largest part of the night holding Tom's hand and praying. I walked with my husband and the Fellow down one more hospital hall to the double doors that led to the surgery suite. I remember that as I kissed Tom good-bye he was relaxed and smiling.

Tom said that as soon as he entered the operating room he saw the surgeon standing at the head of the table. They made small talk briefly with the heart surgeon mentioning that he had done surgery on another Arkansan a few days earlier. Tom answered that he knew the other patient and the doctor laughed about what a small state Arkansas must be for him to have two patients within two weeks of each other who were from another state and actually knew each other. Tom remembers that this operating room was every bit as cold as the other five he had been in. Someone covered his naked body with warm blankets for which he was grateful. He remembers wondering how the doctors worked in such a frigid room although he realized that the cold temperature was for his benefit, meant to help lower his own body temperature as an aid to the surgery. He found himself thinking how difficult the cold must be for the doctors and nurses, and wondering why he had never considered that before. Another IV replaced the saline drip and Tom was under. He remembers nothing else until he awoke that afternoon in the intensive coronary care unit.

I had hoped the waiting room would be nearby, but it was not. I was to wait in the cavernous area I walked through every day going to and from the P to H 11. Once there, I called Ruby and Paul who were at the hospital almost immediately to wait with me. I called our son and our daughter. Then I waited. What a difference this wait was. I was once more surrounded by people-laughing, silent, playing cards, or staring into space, but only two of them were there to support me, to pray on the premises for Tom. I knew prayers for his safety and recovery were going up from many other places. I could feel them and that gave me an indescribable sense of peace and strength. At 12:30 p.m. Tom's surgeon told me that my husband had received a good strong heart. We would later learn that the heart had begun to beat on its own without any stimulation as soon as Tom was taken off the heart-lung machine and blood began flowing through it. I called our son and our daughter to share this miracle we had experienced. We all were, and continue to be, deeply touched that out of some family's loss and deep sorrow we were given a second chance at life together. As our children passed the word on to family and friends, I waited for my first glimpse of my post-transplant husband. Paul and Ruby waited with me a while, praying once more before they left to resume their day. At 1:30 Ash Wednesday afternoon I was allowed into the CVICU to see Tom. My e-mail home to family and friends after the surgery notes that Tom did not require any blood during the surgery and that I still considered him the bravest man I had ever known for facing six heart surgeries so positively.

Our daughter could not get excused from her classes, and would not get to see her father until the following weekend. Tad was not on service at the hospital, but he did have a meeting he had to attend there Wednesday morning after I had called to tell him that his dad was getting a heart. He went to the meeting and when I called to tell him Tom had come through the surgery, he called a couple of doctor friends in Little Rock, friends who had waited previously with him through his dad's surgeries, to tell them the news. He picked up a clean shirt at home, and caught a direct flight from Memphis to Cleveland. By 9:00 that evening Tad was in Tom's room rejoicing because his dad's fingernails were pink for the first time in years. Tom was already laughing and joking. Tom's first memory from the time right after the transplant surgery is of a nurse telling him to open his eyes. He could not. The nurse then said to Tom that he was breathing on his own and that if he would just take a big, deep breath they could pull the ventilator tube. Tom took that breath and shortly thereafter was able to open his eyes, though his focus was still fuzzy from the medicine he had received during surgery. Tad spent the night in my room in the P Building. He had time for one more visit with his father in the morning. As we sat in the waiting room the cell phone in my pocket rang. Oblivious to the rule I was breaking, I answered it at about the same time I saw the *No Cell Phones* sign. I was expecting a call from Leigh about her travel arrangements. It was my intention to answer the call as I quickly left the room; explain to the caller where I was and to hang up. As I stood to do this some poor, stressed member of another family began to yell that my phone was going to kill the patients. For a moment I thought she was going to hit me. Needless to say, my phone was quickly turned off, and apologies were made. I think the level of this woman's anger and the quickness with which she lost control is a great picture of the sort of stress those of us who waited for loved ones to live or to die were under. If she waited without the assurance I felt from the Holy Spirit, I do not know how she managed it alone. Tad, assured that I wasn't about to cause a melee, told his dad he would see him soon, caught a cab to Hopkins Field, and flew home to Memphis, and to his family. By the time Leigh arrived late Friday evening Tom had been moved from the ICU to a room. Here he had his only less than pleasant roommate. This gentleman had occupied the room first and was not happy to have a roommate. We were so elated at Tom's rapid improvement that we hardly acknowledged the churlishness coming from the other side of the room. Leigh, like her brother, noticed that her father's color was once more pink rather than gray. She thought the immediate change nothing short of a miracle. Leigh spent the night with me in the P, giving us a welcome opportunity to catch up on all the news from home. We talked well into the night before falling asleep. Leigh and I grabbed a quick breakfast together; she met some of my friends on the third floor of the P, and she spent more time with her dad before hailing a cab, and catching her flight back to Arkansas.

18

R and R - Recovery and Rehab

Tom spent about a day and a half in the cardiovascular intensive care unit before being moved back to H 11. He remembers looking out the window, no longer at Lake Erie, but at a busy street with snow falling. Post transplant patients were on a different hall from those waiting for organs, so we had a whole new group of care givers, all as professional and as kind as those pre-surgery nurses and aides. One of the nurses was particularly kind to come by late and if Tom was having difficulty getting comfortable enough to sleep, she would give him a back rub to relax his sore and tense muscles. Although Tom expected moving from the transport gurney to his hospital bed to hurt, his chest and ribs seemed particularly sore as he tried to help with the transfer. No doubt the fact that his sternum had been cracked and his ribs spread six times had a lot to do with that. One of Dr. McCarthy's concerns was that the incision through Tom's sternum might not heal well. It was a pleasant surprise for him and for us to see signs of healing very early on. Right after surgery Tom was on fairly large doses of Prednisone, a steroid used in transplant patients; it was making his eyes blurry and his tongue thick. One of his physicians, either the surgeon or the cardiologist, discussed his other medications with him. It was a fairly long list. The anti-rejection drugs given to Tom were Prograf and Celcept. We felt fortunate that he had gotten Prograf rather than Neoral because we had heard that Neoral had more side effects. Actually I think the anti-rejection medications are started during the transplant surgery as an IV. Tom, as a Type II diabetic, was also placed on insulin injections since his

111

endocrine system was fighting off the effects of the surgery as well as the effects of the transplant drugs he needed. The nurses stressed to Tom that he should ask for pain medicine when he *began* to hurt and not to let the pain get a hold on him. They gave him medicine for his discomfort soon after he was settled in his room, but he tried to tough it out, not asking for more when he should have. The pain and the narcotic combined made him very sick to his stomach. Throwing up is not a good thing to experience with a cracked chest. I should also note that Tom still had wires protruding from his chest in case his heart needed to be paced, or as he says, he needed to be *jump started*.

Four days after receiving his new heart, Tom was visited by the transplant physical therapist, Charlie, who introduced himself, visited a moment, and told Tom that he would see him in therapy later that afternoon. Charlie planned to get Tom working on the treadmill. We were certain we had misunderstood, but sure enough, late that afternoon an attendant brought a wheelchair and pushed Tom down the hall and into the elevator, and down another long hall on the tenth floor until we had arrived in Charlie's domain. I had tagged along so that I could learn the route and bring Tom back to the eleventh floor. A couple of the men Tom had known from the pre-transplant side of the floor were already working out. Like little boys, they were anxious to show off how well they were doing. Their treadmills were whirring along at a good clip since they were about two weeks further out from surgery than Tom. Charlie hooked Tom up to several monitors. We got Tom into his Velcro-closure tennis shoes, and he stepped onto one of the treadmills. Charlie started the machine and Tom walked for about five minutes at a snail's pace, but he walked. Elated and exhausted he sank down on a chair. We agree that prior to the transplant he would have been unable to complete even five minutes on a very slow treadmill. When Charlie had monitored Tom's vital signs and felt that he was all right, he allowed me to push him in his wheelchair back to his room.

The weeks following Tom's transplant were in many ways like the weeks before as far as Tom's activities. He still had classes; he could now walk the halls, and was encouraged to do so to increase his stamina. He met the guys he had become friends with as they waited on H 11 in the solarium where they talked, or worked puzzles, or watched movies. One memory is vivid and troubling to Tom. Of the three fellows most often together in the solarium, one was not a believer and was very antagonistic to any conversation that broached the debt both Tom and his friend, Bill, felt to God for their lives. I still came from the P Building to spend most of each day with my husband. As he became stronger, our walks got longer until we were walking down a glass hallway to another building probably one half to a mile distant. I think it was not until he was released from the hospital to join me in the P that he was able to go the whole distance. We were excited finally to be able to complete the walk because there was a wonderful little French café and pastry shop at the end of the hallway. We rewarded ourselves with delicious soups, salads, and sandwiches once we made it down the glass hall.

After heart surgery it was not unusual for Tom's diabetes to flare. It did seem worse after his transplant, probably because of the steroids he was taking to prevent his rejecting his new heart. He was prescribed insulin shots, and I had to learn to give them before he could move to the P Building. Immediately after his surgery Tom was on a long list of medications, all of them typical of what organ recipients were prescribed at that time. One of the side effects of the massive doses of antibiotics he took was that he developed thrush in his mouth, and was then prescribed lozenges and mouthwashes to use several times a day for that. None of these minor problems doused our soaring spirits. The cards, calls and letters from home were as jubilant as we felt. March 12, one week after his transplant, Tom had his first post-transplant heart catheterization and arteriogram to form a base line from which to judge his progress. It was a complete heart catheterization checking both the right and the left sides of the heart. This procedure included coronary arteriography, an intracoronary ultrasound, left ventriculography and a study of intracardiac hemodynamics. At this time Tom also had his first heart biopsy. In this procedure the heart is entered via the jugular vein, and five minuscule snips are retrieved from five areas of the heart to ascertain the rate of rejection. A transplanted organ is treated like any other foreign matter that enters the body in that the body attempts to fight it off as an invader. Tom also had an echocardiogram and withstood the tests well. We were elated when we learned his rejection rate was a *1A*. I felt as if I could quit holding my breath, and that Tom was on the road to recovery. Heart rejection when Tom was a patient at Cleveland Clinic was judged on the following scale: a *0* indicated that your body was totally accepting the donor heart-as good as that sounds, it is not without some pitfalls because it can indicate that your own immune system is so depressed that you may fall prey to other infections and problems; the next level is *1A*, then a *1B*, which bears being more closely monitored. Next is a level *2;* then the last and the worst is a *3. 3* means the patient is in real difficulty, and most likely needs to be hospitalized. On March 13, the cardiologist and surgeon, satisfied with Tom's progress, pulled the ports from his chest and neck. The following day he was released to come live with me in the P Building. I was really quite frightened to be leaving the heart floor and all of the excellent nurses. I know by the time we got Tom settled in our room he was exhausted. His meals were delivered to him from the hospital dietitian which kept me from having to count diabetic exchanges, something I appreciated.

Tom met some of the people I had been telling him about. Paul and Ruby continued to visit as did the young minister from Cleveland Heights. When Tom became a resident of the P, he met two men who had each received a lung transplant on Ash Wednesday when Tom received his heart. We will always wonder if these three were not the beneficiaries of the same donor family. Each day Tom went to physical therapy, and sometimes for other tests as well. One of the side effects of having a transplanted heart showed up first in physical therapy where Tom's heart rate remained high after exercise, rather than slowing down as his original heart would have done. A transplanted heart has no nerve endings connecting it to its body to indicate its proper speed.

About ten days post-transplant Kay, our social worker, told us we could write a note to our donor family. It was hospital policy that we not become personal, ask to meet them, or speak of anything with religious significance or overtones. It was suggested that we choose a suitable card and write a brief note. Think about what a daunting task that was; you cannot just send a grieving family a thank-you note for the organ donation that is allowing you to live. Their loved one is dead and you, someone they have never heard of, are alive because in their most painful hours they did a brave and generous thing. I finally settled on a card and took it back to Tom. Both of us strongly felt that God's hand was in the decision that had resulted in Tom's receiving the particular heart he had been given, but we followed the rules and made no mention of the role our faith was taking or of how it was growing in this whole process. We regret that, because the faith journey we have made is, for us, inseparable from Tom's transplant and the events that both led to and followed it. Tom was too shaky from the prednisone to write legibly, so after we planned what to say together, I wrote the message. We gave the card, sealed in its envelope, to Kay who would take care of mailing it. We were told that most donor families choose not to meet their recipient so we have not been surprised to have never heard from ours. That is their choice, as Tom and I both agree it should be. We do hope that they somehow feel our prayers, and our everlasting gratitude. When we spoke this past year to a group of donor families in our own state I know that in our hearts we were speaking to our donor family as well. Each person we hugged, each person with whom we shared a story or shed tears could have been our own donor family. Old, young, people from every walk of life, they were all generous and brave in their grief, rising above their own loss to do something miraculous for another human being.

On March 19, Tom had his second biopsy and the score for it chilled our souls. He received a *3A*. He was not hospitalized since in effect the P Building was a part of the hospital. He was monitored very closely for the next seven days. Medicines were changed, protocols were tweaked, and Tom was given a big blast of prednisone which, of course, made his vision blurrier and his hands shakier. We were pretty blue that week. When Tom was biopsied again he was found to have a *"Resolving 2"* which meant things were getting better. From that point until this, all of his biopsies have been *0* or *1A*. We have been blessed. At the time Tom received his heart the protocol at The Cleveland Clinic was that for the first four weeks a biopsy was done once a week. The second month post-transplant biopsies were scheduled every two weeks. These tests were moved to four to six weeks apart during months three through ten if all was going well. As the year anniversary approached a biopsy was done every six weeks. The protocol stretched beyond the first year with biopsies required every three to four months for the first three years after transplant. During years four and five biopsies were done four to six months apart. When a heart recipient passed the fifth year anniversary biopsies were no longer regularly scheduled. They were done only if clinically indicated, or on the one-year anniversary of the surgery. After five years a transplant patient was to be seen only twice yearly. At six years out, that is how Tom's appointments are now scheduled.

Tom was growing stronger with each day. Even recuperating from such major surgery his energy level and his color were better than they had been for months prior to the transplant. He made an outing with me to a local grocery store to replenish our pantry. At last the doctor said he was well enough for a celebratory dinner which we enjoyed at one of the great little Italian places in nearby Cleveland Heights. Ready to take on more activity, and tired of the four walls of our room in the P, Tom asked Rose about a museum we had spotted down the street. She said that yes it was very nice, and that it was within walking distance. It was walking distance-about *seven* blocks. By the time we walked there, toured the museum, and walked back facing a good, stiff wind blowing off Lake Erie, we were ready to rest. When Tom's biopsies remained good and were at last spaced two weeks apart, we were released to return to Arkansas. It was April 4. Saying good-bye to people with whom you have walked to the brink of death and back is not easy. Vows are made to stay in touch; some will be kept, but others won't. I left my dishes and the food I had not opened for those still waiting for their transplants. Once more a wheelchair was my luggage trolley as I carted our belongings to the car. As much as I wanted to go home, I was frightened that Tom would become ill on the journey. How would I find a hospital? What would I do? I drove south out of Cleveland in a blowing snow with Tom buckled securely in the passenger seat and our faithful old Mazda slightly less full than it had been in February.

19

Healed but Broken

Between the weather and my concern about how Tom would stand the trip home, it was a tense drive. I do not remember where we spent the night, or when we out ran the snow. I do recall that we had planned to stop at our son's in Memphis, but by the time we were near there, the second day of our travels, we were exhausted and wanted only to get home. A stop would have meant a wait until the children got in from school and Tad got home from the hospital. It would have been well after dark before we got home, and much of our drive would have been in heavier traffic. Tad and Laura would have loved for us to spend the night, but so fresh from the transplant we would have been afraid to do that. We called Tad, trusting him and his family to understand, and knowing they soon would be driving to Arkansas to see how Tom was progressing. As we pulled into our own driveway about two and a half hours later we had a welcoming committee composed of our daughter, our granddaughter and my dad. Our daughter and granddaughter had made a big *Welcome Home* banner and hung it across the carport. It was wonderful to see our loved ones again. Greeting each other emotionally, we went inside where we were surprised by two new purchases for our home. While we were away our daughter had replaced our old refrigerator with a beautiful new one; and our son and his family had replaced our old clothes dryer, the one Tom had rewired numerous times. What a wonderful surprise those were. We put Tom in a recliner to elevate his feet and to rest while Mary and I unloaded the car. We called family and friends that evening to let them know we had arrived safely but we saw none of them for a couple of days. Although we wanted to see people, we had some concerns about Tom's exposure to germs of all sorts. We had left Cleveland with a fairly extensive list of do's and don'ts, most of which related to Tom's suppressed immune system. We could not have a cat; he could not change a diaper-that one did not upset him; he was not to work in a garden with natural fertilizers; he was not to be around mold; some foods that contained live bacteria, like blue cheese, were forbidden; all meats were to be cooked well done. Tom was not to be in crowds, around sniffly, coughing grandchildren (or adults), and he was to be very cautious about shaking hands.

Our first visitors were all from our supper club and *The Board*. Our home had many windows and a circular drive out front. These dear friends called to say they were coming by to see Tom, but would not come in. Their little caravan pulled into our circular drive, and eight or ten of them got out of the cars, and came to stand on the front porch in front of our living room windows. Tom stood in front of the huge, plate glass windows on the inside as I pulled back the curtains. It was grand-kind of like displaying an over-sized baby. They talked through the glass to Tom, smiled, and blew kisses before pulling out into the traffic again.

Not a day had passed in Cleveland when we were not aware of the dire state in which we had left our business. We still did not talk to each other much about it, each trying to protect the other. After his surgery Tom attempted to reach an attorney he had talked with before leaving Arkansas. When he finally got him on the phone, the attorney told Tom that he was in some difficulty due to his dealings with a high profile politician, and that we would have to find another lawyer. Tom renewed his efforts to sell the business and the land on which it was located. He tried briefly to run the business from home as he had done so often in years past when he was ill. He quickly learned that the difficulties the business now faced were going to require more money, more energy, more time than he had to give. He had been told that physically putting himself back in the dust and chemical laden environment of our plant, even though it was OSHA compliant, would be detrimental to his new heart. Tom was not taking money from the business. He was getting a disability check, and I had found a job with a local caterer so that I could eventually have insurance. Our finances were more strained than they had ever been. During this time we invited a group of close friends over one evening for coffee and cake in an effort to thank them for their many kindnesses to us over the past winter. For most of them this was their first real visit with Tom since he had received his new heart. They were amazed at the change in his color and his stamina. One of those friends is a real estate agent. As Tom and she visited that evening she encouraged him to pursue getting a realtor's license. That seemed a good idea to him; it was an idea he says that he had been toying with even while still in Cleveland. He enrolled in a real estate course, passed it, and was hired on her recommendation by the company she was with, a well-established Arkansas firm. She took Tom under her wing and mentored him, giving him invaluable training based on her years of experience.

Tom was making frequent trips back to the Cleveland Clinic for biopsies. For the first several trips every two weeks he used frequent flyer miles we had amassed over the years. I may have flown back once with him, I do not recall. When the frequent flyer miles were used, we paid for airline tickets from our tight budget. When we could no longer do that, I drove with him. Only once did he talk me into letting him make the drive alone, and that was much later in his recovery. We found no avenues of escape from the financial dilemma of our business and on December 18, 2004, the attorney told Tom that it was time to pull the plug. One year to the day from the date we had gone to Cleveland for Tom to be evaluated for a heart transplant, the business filed Chapter 13. It was a strange, strained, and hurtful time. Tom faced it more bravely than I although I am sure he was in agony. The brave front was for my benefit when he was anything but sure of what our next step would be. It must have seemed to him as if his heart and health had been physically mended so his spirit could be broken. I coped by shutting down. We were hosting the annual Christmas dinner for our supper club, the friends who had been with us through all of Tom's heart problems for twenty plus years. The bankruptcy was filed about six hours before dinner was to begin. I was numb. I feared someone would find out. I did not want anyone to criticize Tom. I was embarrassed. I was frightened and dying on the inside, but I did the usual; I put on my make-up, smiled and brightly said *Merry Christmas* though my entire being cried to run and hide. I do not know how we got through that night of lies. It must have been that God was giving us the grace to slowly absorb what had happened to us. I think He led us firmly toward understanding that He was in control; it just didn't happen all at once. We briefly considered filing personal bankruptcy, even filling out the papers. When Tom went to the courthouse to actually file, someone, an officer of the court, I suppose, told him that would not be necessary. It is awful to watch all that you have worked for slip away. Yes, some of our problems rested squarely on our shoulders for poor decisions we had made; more of what happened to us happened because of the severity of Tom's illness the year prior to his transplant. I know Tom must have wanted to give up, but he never said that; he never quit trying to find solutions. Of all the things that happened during this time, the thing that hurt me most was that my ninety-year-old father was told by a relative about the bankruptcy. Dad had quit reading the paper and was not in great health. I had wanted more than anything to protect him from the knowledge of what had happened. Dad had been a good, hard working business man, a child of the Great Depression, who had raised me to be a better manager than I had been. The knowledge that he would be disappointed in me ate at my heart. In all honesty, my pride, I am sure, was involved in not wanting him to find out, and I did not want him to think ill of Tom. To my father's everlasting credit all he said to me was that he knew what had happened. There was never a word of disappointment or blame aimed at Tom or myself. Dad had been a silent partner in the business, and had invested in it over the years. He knew how much we were hurting, and he loved us too much to add to our pain. My dad sure wasn't perfect, but he taught me a lot about unconditional love.

As we struggled through the holiday season and into the New Year with Tom still attempting to sell real estate, I started a new job in a medical office where my working conditions were better, and where I would be able to obtain benefits and good insurance. As seemed to be the case in our lives at this time, for every positive thing that happened, there seemed to be an opposing blow. We were unable to find a way out of the morass of problems we had. The crowning horror was that because during the latter stages of Tom's heart disease we had borrowed against our home to keep the business running, we learned that the banks planned to foreclose, not only on the land where the business was located, but also on our home. Unbeknownst to either of us, a cousin, an attorney in Florida, made multiple trips to Arkansas at his own expense in an effort to intervene. Alan was unsuccessful. I descended into some sort of hell, and I do not know how I continued to function. I think I would have been physically ill if I had been forced to join my husband on the courthouse steps as the clerk sold our property to the bank. Tom faced that alone, a fact which shames me. The bank gave us a deadline for moving out. Our daughter and granddaughter no longer lived with us, but there was still my father to consider. Tom and I worried about what this would do to him. We began looking for places to buy or to rent. There wasn't much money to go around. As a realtor Tom worked on a commission. He had not had the time to build up a clientele. We decided that we could not buy; the things we could afford to rent, we did not like. We were almost ready just to take the next thing we saw regardless of where or what it was if it was clean, and had bedrooms enough for the three of us. Tom had worked with a couple of young women about our daughter's age since he had been in real estate. They worked for a mortgage company that he and his partner often used with the homes they sold. One day the two of them, who knew the story of Tom's heart transplant and our efforts to start over, told him that they would like to buy our house from the bank as an investment. They would allow us to live there for a year, giving us enough time to find something else. Again the Lord put people in our path at just the right time. These modern day good Samaritans had known Tom for less than a year; they had never met me. What made them do this? We were astounded. I remember thinking it was just too good to be true, but it was. Their kindness may have meant more to me than to Tom because I did not have to hurriedly uproot my father. I knew that was going to be a difficult experience for him at the very best, but to have torn him in six weeks or less from the little house that had become his home would have been heart wrenching.

If our friends realized the extent of our plight, they were kind enough to pretend that they did not. Tom and I were learning to handle adversity together by being more open with each other. We were learning not to place blame. We were learning to be kinder and more loving. God used this time in a mighty way to grow us and to strengthen our marriage. In spite of the precariousness of our situation, it was, in some ways, a good time. Tom's health was better than it had been in years. I enjoyed my new job. Tom was still learning the ropes in real estate. He, even then, was trying to convince himself that if he just tried harder, put more of himself into it, he would enjoy it, but he didn't. After about eighteen frustrating months Tom admitted that he doubted he would ever be a great realtor. He had thought he could sell anything since he had been a successful salesman of technical products, but it just was not working out.

He had a couple of clients he was working with, and one of them thought he and his family would like country living. Tom had taken them to several areas and had not found just the right thing when someone told him about a road in the far western reaches of our county where some nice homes were being constructed. The weekend weather was pretty so he asked me to drive with him to find this place. We looked and looked without finding what he thought had been described to him. We did, on our drive, discover a smaller home with a huge yard enclosed by a wood and stone fence. It had a *For Sale by Owner* sign out front, and there was a car in the driveway. The car belonged to the owner who was there doing some chores. When Tom got out of our car and talked to her she indicated that she would be willing to work with him if his client was interested. Tom thought the house was probably smaller than his client wanted but with the fence and fruit trees in the yard it was an attractive place. Since our search for anything else had been unsuccessful, Tom decided he would at least tell his client about the place. As we pulled out of the drive we stopped to get a flyer from the tube by the owner's sign. Looking back at the broad lawn and the little house, I told Tom that I just loved it. I am a city girl born and bred, so that is certainly not what he had expected to hear from me. Our lives had been so stressful for so long that I think the idea of the quiet of living in such a place really appealed to me. We talked about the property all the way back to town, concluding that there was no way we could afford a house and thirteen acres. Tom planned to show it to his client within the week, and I planned to forget about it, thinking that I was probably romanticizing the whole idea of country living anyway.

Tom was right. His client did not want a home that small. Actually, he had determined that he really did not want to live in the country at all and now had Tom showing him houses in the city. Tom and I could not get the little brown house in the country out of our minds. Tom says that he started to pray that if it was part of the Lord's plan for us to be in that house that He would show us a way to do it. I had been praying, and continued to pray for a good place for us and my dad. There did not seem to be anything on the horizon. I think we even drove back to the country to look at the place again. Finally, Tom, tired of being tantalized by the hope of obtaining it, called the owner and asked if she would have time for a cup of coffee. Over that cup of coffee Tom told her our story. He asked if she would consider a graduated lease with it becoming a lease-purchase plan. To his surprise she said that she would think about it and get back to him. They talked several more times. I am sure she investigated our background. Why would she trust two people whose resources were so limited? Why would she believe that we would make our payments and take care of her investment? I cannot say with certainty that in her place I would have believed us, but she did. We can think of no reason why she did, other than God's hand was in this. It was His plan to help restore us, and He helped choose this haven for us.

Not only did the owner agree to our lease-purchase idea, she agreed to let us do some minor re-decorating before we moved in. She still had a few things stored in the garage that she wanted to get, but she gave us keys. The house was in immaculate condition and we could have moved in immediately, but we changed some interior paint colors and removed some wallpaper. We went out evenings after work and on weekends, and did the work ourselves. The young people who had bought our house in town put it on the market. For a while there were no successful offers on it so we were not rushed. We often took my father with us when we went to the country to work trying to accustom him to the upcoming move. He liked the brown house with its front porch and back deck. He enjoyed being where there was a garden and wildlife, but he, as many older people do, became confused about exactly where we were. He often told people that we were moving him up close to the Missouri line. I am sure that the drive through the mountains west of town reminded him of roads he had traveled as a younger man. I know the move was hard for him although he chose to go with us rather than to get an apartment in town. For any difficulty we caused him, I am genuinely sorry. By autumn the three of us were in our new home.

Tom was still unhappily trying to sell real estate. One day as I listened to his complaints about his job, I asked him if he was so miserable why he didn't put his education to work and find a teaching job. Tom had never been one to either complain or to give up, and I did not like what I was hearing from him. I suspect more to show me up than for any other reason, he picked up the phone and called the local two-year community college to ask if they were hiring. He spoke to the Science Dean who became more interested as Tom explained that he had an undergraduate degree in math and physics and a Master's Degree in Physics. Tom told the Dean that he had no experience in teaching except that he had once been a flight instructor, and that when one of the local private high schools found themselves with a class full of students wanting to take computer assisted drafting and, at the last minute, no one to teach the course, Tom had taught the CAD course. As the conversation went on, the Dean asked Tom where he lived and how quickly could he get to the campus for an interview. Tom thought he could be there in under a half hour so the Dean agreed to wait for him. When Tom arrived he was interviewed by the Dean and the Chairmen of the Physical Science and Chemistry Departments. He was hired that afternoon, and he has been teaching for several years. We are sure God gave him a nudge in that direction. Things simply fell into place too swiftly and too smoothly for there to be another answer. Tom has found that he is good at teaching; he likes the challenge of saying the right words to create an *ah-ha* moment when a student gets it.

So is this our fairy tale ending? Do we live happily ever after? I don't really believe in fairy tales anymore. We know not all stories have a happy ending. We know that sometimes *happy* and *joy* are not the same. We are quite sure that our story will have a joyful ending, and that however it ends, it is in God's hands.

20

A Changed Heart

Two people can travel the same road at the same time and still not see the same sights on the journey; especially if they are viewing their surroundings through different lenses. That is what happened to Tom and me. Tom will tell you that I am a stronger, older believer than he, but I am not sure his assessment is true. I have been a believer for a very long time, but my faith journey has been a crooked one, sometimes more full of detours than of any real advances. I was influenced by a mother and wonderful Sunday school teachers who grounded me early in God's love. I have been blessed by family and friends who have unselfishly shared both their love and the love of Christ with me. I had my own moment when I knew without a doubt that my life was out of control, and I could do nothing to fix it long before Tom had such a moment in his own life. I knew in that moment that the *lonely* child need never be lonely again; that the Holy Spirit was real; that He was there for me and that although I could turn away from Him, He would not turn from me, nor would He let me go. There is a contemporary Christian song I love that says *you cannot fall below His resting arms.* I know that is true.

Tom, on the road we shared, looked through a different lens. He tried so hard to steer a straight course, to be a good husband, a good dad, a good friend. He worked hard at those things and tried desperately to control anything that might pose a threat to those relationships. Sometimes he succeeded. After Tom received his new heart so many things in our lives were still in a downward spiral that it would have been easy for Tom to ask the Lord what he had been saved for. A faith not well founded and much exercised can prove hard to hold onto in adversity. Tom and I had grown up in different Protestant denominations. In our life as a couple we attended and left churches in each one of them. In each church we met strong believers and made deep friendships. Each church helped us clarify what we were seeking. My husband began to talk with me about returning to an evangelical church we had once attended. It was a church where we had enjoyed strong Bible teaching, one where we felt we had been encouraged to have a closer relationship to Jesus Christ. We went back to that congregation and had not been there long when we took a course that encouraged exploring one's beliefs; in fact the name of the course was *Explore,* and it was led by the teaching pastor who had so many years before stood by Tom's hospital bed in the ICU and prayed for Tom and *Sarah.* The course lasted several weeks and was fairly intense with a good bit of reading and questions to answer. Tom says this course had a greater impact on his life than anything else he had ever heard. He says that he finally got it. Tom and I have shared our story with his recording the words, and with my doing the writing for us both. I think his final statement about a changed heart is best said in Tom's own words.

"I recognized that God was in control," Tom says. "He had a hand in what we were doing and has ultimately given us a happier and more peaceful life." Tom says, "I wandered through life and through my experiences in churches trying to be good on my own. I just didn't get it. In this course, this teacher laid it on the line in a way that made me realize that God was in control. I could finally see what I had been missing by trying to be in complete control of every aspect of my own life. It was not a mountain top experience; it was as if someone had rapped me on the head." Tom's father used to say that a certain mule he owned would work pretty well once you got his attention, but you had to tap him on the head with a stout stick to get his attention. God had Tom's attention at last. Tom continues, "All of a sudden I realized my life was changing. I was less angry, less hostile toward people. I could see that by losing everything, I had gained everything-my life, my family, my *everything.* It is hard to explain, but what I gained was God. I had worked so hard at being a good husband, a good father, a good provider, but it was all about me and what I could do. I held, or tried to hold, total control and I felt slighted if anyone questioned me or my motives. God used our circumstances to discipline me, to teach me, to test me and to give me a second, and a third, and more chances, and to draw me to Himself. I fought with Him and in so doing I lost my financial footing, my business, our home; there were times I almost lost my marriage, and ultimately I came close to losing my life. I was a loser, a spiritual phony, yet God in His bountiful mercy saved me. I do not know why. Life is not perfect; I am not perfect, but God is, and with Him in control the road is so much easier. Perhaps He saved me so I can tell my story. He changed my heart."

LaVergne, TN USA
12 July 2010
189302LV00002B/204/P